DATE DUE

3-8

From Cognitive-Behavior Therapy
to Psychotherapy Integration

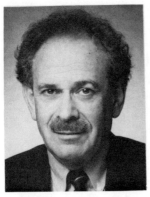

Marvin R. Goldfried, PhD, is Professor of Psychology and Psychiatry at the State University of New York at Stony Brook. In addition to his teaching, clinical supervision, and research, he maintains a limited practice of psychotherapy in New York City. He is a diplomate in clinical psychology, editorial board member of professional journals, and author of several books. Dr. Goldfried is cofounder of the Society for the Exploration of Psychotherapy Integration.

Other books by Marvin R. Goldfried

Rorschach Handbook of Clinical and Research Applications
(with G. Stricker and I.B. Weinder)

Behavior Change Through Self-Control
(with M. Merbaum)

Clinical Behavior Therapy
(with G.C. Davison)

Converging Themes in Psychotherapy: Trends in Psychodynamic, Humanistic, and Behavioral Practice

Handbook of Psychotherapy Integration
(with J.C. Norcross)

From Cognitive-Behavior Therapy to Psychotherapy Integration

An Evolving View

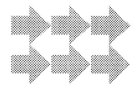

Marvin R. Goldfried, PhD

 Springer Publishing Company

To Anita,

my companion in change

Springer Publishing Company, Inc.
536 Broadway
New York, NY 10012-3955

Cover design by Tom Yabut
Production Editor: Joyce Noulas

95 96 97 98 99 / 5 4 3 2 1

Library of Congress Cataloging-in-Publication Data

Goldfried, Marvin R.
    From cognitive-behavior therapy to psychotherapy integration : an evolving view / Marvin R. Goldfried.
       p.   cm. —(Springer series on behavior therapy and behavioral medicine)
    Includes bibliographical references and index.
    ISBN 0-8261-8780-3
    1. Cognitive therapy.   2. Behavior therapy.   3. Eclectic psychotherapy.   I. Title.   II. Series: Springer series on behavior therapy and behavioral medicine (unnumbered)
RC489.C63G65   1995
    616.89'142—dc20   CIP 94-39953

Printed in the United States of America

Contents

Permissions

Chapters 2-15 in this book originally appeared in the following publications and are reprinted with permission. These chapters are here published in modified form from their original sources.

Chapter 2 is adapted from Goldfried, M. R., & Pomeranz, D. M. (1968). "The role of assessment and behavior modification," *Psychological Reports*, 23, 75-87. Copyright © 1968 by *Psychological Reports*.

Chapter 3 is adapted from Goldfried, M. R., & Kent, R. N. (1972). "Traditional versus behavioral personality assessment: A comparison of methodological and theoretical assumptions." *Psychological Bulletin*, 77, 409-420. Copyright © 1972 by the American Psychological Association.

Chapter 4 is adapted from Goldfried, M. R. (1987). "Assessment of cognitive activities" in J. P. Dauwalder, M. Perrez, & V. Hobi (Eds.), *Annual Controversial Issues in Behavior Modification*. Berwyn, PA: Swets North America. Copyright © 1987 by Swets North America.

Chapter 5 is adapted from Goldfried, M. R. (1971). "Systematic desensitization as training in self-control," *Journal of Consulting and Clinical Psychology*, 37, 228-234. Copyright © 1971 by the American Psychological Association.

Chapter 6 is adapted from Goldfried, M. R. (1988). "The application of rational restructuring to anxiety disorders," *Counseling Psychologist*, 16, 50-68. Copyright © 1988 by the Division of Counseling Psychology.

Preface

In a sense, behavior therapy and I grew up together. I have been involved with behavior therapy at the State University of New York at Stony Brook since the mid-1960s, when this new approach to intervention was just beginning to gain a footing within therapeutic circles. Since that time, much of my teaching, clinical supervision, research, and writing has dealt with the expanding scope of behavior therapy. During these past 25 years, my clinical writings have focused on a number of issues, including behavioral assessment and case formulation, the relevance of cognitive variables for behavioral interventions, the view of behavior therapy as training in coping skills, and the integration of contributions from other orientations into behavior therapy. In tandem with my own thinking, the behavior therapy of the 1960s moved toward cognitive-behavior therapy in the 1970s, and has been moving toward interest in psychotherapy integration since the 1980s.

As a psychotherapy orientation, behavior therapy is uniquely advantaged, in that its growth and development have been nurtured by both clinical observation and research contributions. Clinical practice has provided behavior therapy with the context of discovery, and subsequent research has served as the context of verification, attempting to confirm and clarify what was initially observed clinically. As any practicing therapist well knows, clinical observations typically occur well in advance of what one reads in the research literature. To the extent that therapists are in good contact with clinical reality, they are influenced by the corrective experiences intrinsic to their clinical work. In many ways Skinner was right: we as therapists are "shaped" by our clients, who reinforce those interventions that work, and extinguish those that do not.

As a result of both the research literature and attempts to apply behavior therapy in a clinical setting, behavior therapy has become more cognitive in nature. In addition, the behavioral orientation recognizes the importance of the therapeutic relationship, has encouraged clients in the development of coping skills, and has taken into account the relevance of the interpersonal system. Most recently, there is the beginning recognition of the role of affect in therapy and the importance of acknowledging potential contributions that other orientations might make.

In the introductory chapter written especially for this book, together with the sampling of my writings over the past 25 years, the emphasis has been primarily on clinical and conceptual issues that have moved my view of the change process from behavior therapy to that of psychotherapy integration. With this very distinct clinical focus, it is hoped that this collection will be of interest to practicing clinicians and graduate students struggling to learn more about therapeutic change. Given the current interest in psychotherapy integration, this volume has relevance not only to behaviorally-oriented clinicians, but to therapists of other orientations as well.

Acknowledgments

The growth and development of many of the ideas expressed in this book would not have been possible without the support and encouragement of numerous colleagues and students over the years. I am particularly grateful to my friends and associates in the Society for the Exploration of Psychotherapy Integration—SEPI—who have helped me to better understand the depth and breadth of therapeutic change. Acknowledgment also needs to be made to the patients with whom I have worked over the years, who, because they did not always change in the way they were "supposed" to, led me to question the accuracy of my concepts and the efficacy of my methods.

The original idea for compiling the collection of my papers came from my colleague and frequent lunch companion, Windy Dryden, to whom I am indebted. Some of the material that has been included in this book is based on the work done together with students and colleagues over the years, without whose insights and efforts these papers would never have been written. For their collaboration, I would like to gratefully acknowledge the contributions of Louis Castonguay, Windy Dryden, Adele Hayes, Ronald Kent, David Pomeranz, and Clive Robins.

I would also like to thank Cecily Osley for her dedication and hard work associated with preparing the manuscript, and to Anna Samoilov for her invaluable editorial assistance. Work on this book was also greatly facilitated by grant #15044 from the National Institute of Mental Health.

Finally, my very deep and sincere appreciation needs to be expressed to my family, which has served as both a safe home base and as an important impetus for change. I would like to acknowledge the support of my sons, Dan and Mike, whose growth and development over the past two decades have provided me with an ongoing inspiration for renewal. And finally, my loving thanks goes to my wife Anita — my companion in change — to whom this book is dedicated.

Part I
INTRODUCTION

The progress of science is the work of creative minds. Every creative mind that contributes to scientific advances works, however, within two limitations. It is limited, first, by ignorance, for one discovery waits upon that other which opens the way to it. Discovery and its acceptance are, however, limited also by the habits of thought that pertain to the culture of any region and period, that is to say, by the *Zeitgeist*: an idea too strange or preposterous to be thought in one period of western civilization may be readily accepted as true only a century or two later.

E.G. Boring

This book is about change. It deals not only with how we are able to help our clients to change, but also about how we, their therapists, have evolved in our own thinking and practice. Wachtel (1985), a psychodynamic therapist who has written about the rapprochement across different theoretical orientations, has captured the essence of the change process among therapists by suggesting: "If your theoretical perspective has remained constant throughout your career, it's a good sign that you've been looking at too narrow a range of data" (p. 16). Like our clients, some therapists deal with change more willingly than others. Some, the "true believers," never depart from what they originally were taught.

Harry Stack Sullivan once suggested that people are more human than otherwise. Although he was referring to his patients at the time, he might just as well have been speaking about his colleagues. And since therapeutic schools of thought are developed and perpetuated by individuals, any understanding of the change process among patients can help to shed light on how we, as therapists, may be able to extend our conceptual and behavioral boundaries. Just as our patients

1

at times have difficulty in thinking and acting in ways that might help improve their lives, so do we, their therapists, often restrict ourselves in ways that may limit our clinical effectiveness.

Our clients enter therapy because the cognitive, emotional, and behavioral patterns that may have originally helped them to adjust to the reality of their life are no longer working for them. Similarly, an increasing number of therapists have been considering the possibility of expanding their theoretical orientations, as the ones that they have originally been taught do not always work for them clinically. With the pressures associated with managed healthcare, the growing sophistication of consumers of psychotherapy, and the competition from biological psychiatry, there seems to be a greater motivation for therapists to change.

1

The Growth and Development of Cognitive-Behavior Therapy

This chapter and those that follow provide an account of some of the changes that have occurred within the practice of clinical behavior therapy over the last 25 years. In many respects, behavior therapy and I grew up together professionally. Although my original orientation in graduate school was psychodynamic in nature, I began to learn about behavior therapy in the early 1960s, upon arriving at Stony Brook. This behavioral orientation gradually evolved into one that recognized the importance of cognition, and eventually to one that has become more open to contributions from other theoretical orientations. Having a scientist-practitioner identity in action as well as in ideology served as an ongoing motivation for me to think about and justify what I was doing clinically. There is also something about demonstrating behavior therapy behind a one-way mirror, and standing up in front of a class of graduate students year after year to justify one's therapeutic behavior, that fosters such an ongoing reevaluation.

The grounding I have had in the scientist-practitioner model has motivated me to integrate clinical observations with research findings. As a graduate student in the 1950s, when projective techniques were all the rage, I found it difficult to take on faith some of the accepted clinical lore. What was the evidence, for example, that confirmed the interpretation of certain responses on the Rorschach, such as the perception of things at a distance (i.e., vista responses) being indicative of subjects' ability to obtain a perspective on themselves? This

3

prompted me to carry out research on projective techniques, to test out the validity of such interpretations (e.g. Goldfried, Stricker, & Weiner, 1971).

My involvement in both clinical and research work also led me to appreciate how it was often the case where *clinical practice* provided a more accurate picture of reality than did research findings. For example, there was a time in the 1960s when the research literature came to the erroneous conclusion that relaxation training was not a viable clinical intervention unless it was used within the context of systematic desensitization. Inasmuch as our clients do not read the research literature, they are in an excellent position to provide us with a more unbiased perspective on clinical phenomena. They behave in ways that have nothing to do with current trends in the field, and will change or not change because we have managed to come up with the optimal intervention, regardless of whether the methods we use happen to be fashionable at the time.

There are many such lessons that clients have taught us as cognitive-behavior therapists. It became evident with the attempt to apply behavior therapy in clinical practice that it was simply not possible to do so without an adequate assessment and precise clinical formulation. Practicing behavior therapists also learned that cognitive variables often played a crucial role in both the assessment and intervention procedures. It also became apparent that although clients might change their behavior as a function of our interventions, they would not always cognitively process their therapeutic gains. Indeed, they often "yes-butted" the changes that they made. And in more recent years, an increasing number of cognitive-behavior therapists have come to the conclusion that their orientation might not be adequate to handle all cases that they encountered clinically, and that concepts and methods from psychodynamic and experiential orientations might at times prove to be helpful.

The greater willingness of cognitive-behavior therapists, and indeed clinicians of other orientations, to cross theoretical boundaries is particularly interesting in light of the long tradition that therapists have had in stereotyping each other. For example, behavior therapists have often been viewed as cold, calculating, and manipulative; psychodynamic therapists have been seen as aloof, woolly-headed, and overly speculative; and experiential therapists have been perceived as "touchy-feely," anti-intellectual, and indeed nonthinking. The pejorative labels we have applied to clinicians of other orientations have helped us to retain our very clear sense of identity, as well as the belief that we have the inside track on truth and efficacy. Unfortunately, it has also prevented us from complementing our own clinical limitations with what might be the strengths of other orientations.

That cognitive-behavior therapists, as well as psychodynamic therapists, have been extending their horizons is confirmed in a study carried out by Friedling, Goldfried, and Stricker (1984). In a survey of professionals who obtained their doctorates in clinical psychology from either a behaviorally-oriented program (i.e., SUNY at Stony Brook) or a psychoanalytically-oriented one (i.e., Adelphi University), a considerable amount of theoretical overlap was found on the activities endorsed in a practice questionnaire. Seventy-eight percent of the psychodynamic practices and 55 percent of the behavioral procedures were reported as being used by both orientations. Clearly, these professionals were not strictly adhering to the orientations they learned in graduate school.

Although many of the cognitive-behavioral methods that were developed in the 1960s continue to be viable, there have been changes in the cognitive-behavior therapy of the 1990s (Goldfried & Castonguay, 1993; Goldfried & Davison, 1994). Originally advocating that clients' behavior should be viewed as being specific to a given set of circumstances, cognitive-behavior therapists now have a greater recognition of consistencies of behavior—especially interpersonal patterns—that need to be dealt with during therapy. Clearly moving in a direction that appears to be more psychodynamic in nature, cognitive-behavior therapists are also acknowledging the importance of the therapist-client relationship itself as a potential sample of clients' difficulties, and a useful vehicle for implementing therapeutic change. There is also more attention being paid to systemic contributions, whereby marital and family interventions are being considered as being important both to bring about and maintain change over time. Finally, as both the cognitive-behavioral orientation and those individuals who practice within it have evolved and matured, there has been an acknowledgement that not all problems are equally amenable to change. Thus, both therapists and their clients need to accept the realistic limitations to the change process, particularly with longstanding problems that do not easily lend themselves to change (e.g., those based on early and severe abuse).

FROM BEHAVIOR THERAPY TO
COGNITIVE-BEHAVIOR THERAPY

Although psychodynamic theory and therapy was the original frame-work within which I was trained in graduate school, there was also a very strong emphasis on learning. And while the gap between psycho-dynamic therapy and learning theory was indeed a large one, Dollard and Miller's (1950) classic book *Personality and Psychotherapy* pro-vided an important mediator between the two. By translating psycho-dynamic therapy into learning theory terminology, I found it rela-tively easy to adopt a behaviorally oriented approach to clinical work in the 1960s. Indeed, many of the basics of what was to become be-havior therapy are noted in Dollard and Miller's classic work, some of which are described in Chapter 12 of this book. Also of particular in-terest is the fact that Dollard and ·Miller's work was a bridge that went both ways, and has been acknowledged by Wachtel (1977) as helping him to understand how behavior therapy might usefully be incorpo-rated into psychodynamic therapy.

Another important influence in my thinking was an article by Breger and McGaugh in 1965, in which they critiqued behavior ther-apy by stating that in its attempt to extrapolate learning principles from the laboratory into the clinic setting, only notions of operant and classical conditioning were recognized. They noted that the cog-nitively-oriented work in learning had been totally ignored and conse-quently represented a very definite shortcoming of behavior therapy. The reactions of my colleagues and myself to their critique were im-mediately negative. My own interpretation of this article was that it was motivated by the desire to have the contributions of Edward Tolman placed on an equal par with those of Ivan Pavlov and B. F. Skinner. A year or two afterwards, as we began to gain some perspec-tive on their contribution, it became apparent that Breger and McGaugh were pointing out that if behavior therapy were to be based on learning, then it needed to take into account the field of cognitive psychology, which was just beginning to emerge at the time.

In 1968, some of my colleagues and I organized a symposium for the meetings of the American Psychological Association, entitled "Cognitive processes in behavior modification." The participants con-sisted of Gerald C. Davison, Thomas J. D'Zurilla, Gordon L. Paul, Stuart Valins, and myself; Louis Breger served as discussant. Arriving at the conclusion that behavior therapy needed to incorporate cognitive constructs in both its assessment and treatment procedures, the purpose of the symposium stated the following:

> The predominant conceptualization of the "Behavior Therapies" as conditioning techniques involving little or no cognitive influence on behavior change is questioned. It is suggested that current procedures should be modified and new procedures developed to capitalize upon the human organism's unique capacity for cognitive control.

Cognitive psychology was in its very early stages of development in the 1960s, and the primary impetus for the development of techniques associated with cognitive-behavior therapy came much more from a clinical need. Although desensitization was found to be very effective clinically, there were instances where one could readily observe that cognitively mediated anxiety undermined its effectiveness. Consequently, the recognition that cognitive constructs might play a useful role in behavior therapy occurred without benefit of the empirical basis that had been used in the development of intervention methods having their origins in classical or operant conditioning. Nonetheless, there were many behavior therapists who were in good contact with clinical reality, and recognized that the conditioning models were incomplete.

In the inaugural issue of the journal *Behavior Therapy*, Bergin (1970), an advocate of the need to develop an eclectic approach to psychotherapy, applauded the movement to introduce cognitive procedures into behavior therapy. In commenting on this interest in cognition, he made a most astute observation:

> The sociological and historical importance of the movement should not be underestimated, for it has three important consequences. It significantly reduces barriers to progress due to narrow school allegiances, it brings the energies of a highly talented and experimentally sophisticated group to bear upon the intricate and often baffling problems of objectifying and managing the subjective, and it underscores the notion that a pure behavior therapy does not exist. (Bergin, 1970, p. 207)

Bergin was quite accurate in his forecast of the impact that the introduction of cognitive variables into behavior therapy might make. Many of the behavior therapists who became involved in the cognitive-behavior therapy movement (e.g., Davison, Goldfried, Lazarus, Mahoney, Meichenbaum) later on moved to develop an interest in psychotherapy integration.

Starting with the notion that it was important to attend to what clients were "telling themselves" soon led practicing cognitive-behavior therapists to recognize that their clients would not always be able to report on any coherent self-statements. Quite often, however, they would acknowledge that they were behaving "as if" they were saying certain things to themselves. It became apparent that our difficulties in eliciting cognitive mediators may have been more of a function of our incorrect conceptualization of the nature of the "internal dialogue," rather than simply our faulty attempts to do so. Instead, what cognitive-behavior therapists needed to attend to was the *meaning* that clients assigned to situations or people, however implicit it might be. Although cognitive-behavior therapists rarely spoke of "unconscious processes" in the psychodynamic sense, they more readily embraced the "schema" construct from cognitive psychology. What is particularly fascinating is that psychodynamic therapists were similarly—but independently—drawing on the cognitive sciences, recognizing that the notion of "schema" captured the phenomena that they were grappling with clinically.

THE INTEREST IN PSYCHOTHERAPY INTEGRATION

In order to move from the competitive, indeed adversarial relationship among different approaches to therapy, a common ground is needed. Not only can such a common ground provide a useful platform on which to dialogue with each other, it also may help us as therapists to obtain a better understanding of the clinical change process. Thus, rather than discussing change with each other in terms of either abstract theoretical constructs or specific techniques, a more intermediate level of abstraction—the therapeutic strategy or principle—might represent both a convenient and significant place to begin. As I have suggested elsewhere:

> To the extent that clinicians of varying orientations are able to arrive at a common set of strategies, it is likely that what emerges will consist of robust phenomena, as they have managed to survive the dis-

tortions imposed by the therapists's varying theoretical biases. (Goldfried, 1980a, p. 996)

In reviewing what therapists of differing orientations have described as being central to the change process within their own particular orientation, it is possible to extract some common themes that seem to cut across these different vantage points (Goldfried & Padawer, 1982). These common therapeutic principles include: (1) The presence of expectations that psychotherapy will be helpful; (2) the availability of an optimal therapeutic relationship; (3) the use of feedback for purposes of increasing patients' awareness; (4) the facilitation of corrective experiences; and (5) the opportunity to engage in ongoing reality testing.

Expectation that Therapy Will Help

Frank (1961), one of the earliest writers in the field to advocate the existence of common factors across the different orientations, has maintained that providing positive expectations to patients who are otherwise demoralized plays a pivotal role in the change process. Although many would agree that the facilitation of hope can have a positive therapeutic impact, it is generally acknowledged that more is required in therapy than a promissory note that the treatment is going to be helpful. In short, it is an important necessary, but not sufficient condition for change.

An Optimal Therapeutic Relationship

In his writing about the change process, Rogers (1957) suggested that the therapeutic relationship itself was *the* central component of how change occurred. Although there certainly may be important therapeutic benefits to an ongoing interaction with a warm, emotionally attuned and genuine therapist—indeed the therapeutic relationship has been found to be an important predictor of therapeutic success—most contemporary therapists would conclude that it, too, is necessary but not always sufficient.

In writing about the therapeutic relationship, behavior therapists have typically described it as the "nonspecific" aspects of change. It has been referred to as such not because the characteristics of a good therapeutic relationship could not be identified, but more because it was not specified within the theoretical framework at the time. However, extrapolating from a psychodynamic framework, Bordin (1979) has provided a model of the therapeutic alliance that is useful to clinicians of all orientations, including cognitive-behavior therapists. Bordin suggests that the therapeutic alliance is made up of three factors. The first is the therapeutic *bond* between therapist and client, which might be thought of as the "chemistry" between them. Thus, clients perceive their therapists as caring, understanding, and knowledgeable, and therapists view their client as someone with whom they can work clinically. In addition to the bond, the alliance is also comprised of an agreement between both client and therapist on the *goals* of the therapy (e.g., symptom reduction, improvement in interpersonal relations). As we all unhappily know from clinical experience, a poor alliance may result when we and our clients work at cross purposes. The final aspect of the therapeutic alliance consists of an agreement between client and therapist on the *means* by which the goals may be accomplished. Although the goals and means may vary from orientation to orientation, agreement is central to a successful clinical outcome.

Helping Clients to Become More Aware

In viewing this third aspect of the therapeutic change process from an information-processing perspective, we might suggest that the role of the therapist is to help clients "redeploy their attention" to aspects of their functioning about which they may not be aware, such as their feelings, thoughts, motivations, or actions. Thus, our clients may not be aware of connections between their thinking and their feelings, between their feelings and their behavior, the effect that others have on them, or the impact their actions have on others. Based on their past learning, clients' views of themselves and others may be inaccurate, and this inaccurate model of the world can cause problems in their lives. This aspect of the change process involves helping them to see things more accurately; it is the "cognitive" aspect of cognitive-behavior therapy.

Encouragement in Corrective Experiences

This is the "risk-taking" component of therapeutic change, and reflects the "behavioral" aspect of cognitive-behavior therapy (e.g., exposure). It also can be seen in the writings of Alexander and French

(1946), who suggest that it is important for patients to behave in ways that they may have been reluctant or afraid to in the past, so that they can experience that the consequences were not nearly so negative — and might even be favorable.

The corrective experience is at the very core of therapeutic change. Leading authorities within the cognitive-behavioral, psychodynamic and experiential orientations have described the corrective experience as being "basic," "crucial," and "essential" to therapeutic change (Brady et al., 1980). What seems to differ from school to school is the venue in which the corrective experience occurs. In cognitive-behavior therapy, it tends to occur *between* sessions, when clients take such interpersonal risks as those involving self-assertion, or behaving in ways that help reduce their phobic avoidance. In psychodynamic and experiential therapies, the corrective experience is more likely to take place *within* the session itself, by virtue of the therapist reacting in an accepting rather than aversive way to the client's new ways of acting, thinking, or emotional expression.

Ongoing Reality Testing

Helping patients to engage in ongoing reality testing essentially involves the two previous principles, in that they become more aware of certain aspects of themselves and others and take risks as a result of this new awareness. This cognitive and behavioral process helps facilitate an ongoing cycle of further awareness and risk-taking. Much like the psychodynamic concept of "working through," the synergistic interaction between insight and action helps patients to become aware that things might now be different in their lives, which is then confirmed by actual corrective experiences.

Delineating common principles of change in no way implies that therapists from different orientations do the same thing. Quite the contrary. Because behavioral, psychodynamic, and experiential therapies have their original roots in different sets of determinants — behavior, thinking, and emotion — there has been a differential emphasis in their unique contributions. Reflecting its background in experimental psychology, behavior therapy has developed methods for establishing graded tasks that can increase the likelihood that clients will engage in behavioral risk-taking. Psychodynamic therapy has become sensitive to implicit meaning structures present in patients, particularly as they may play themselves out within the context of the therapeutic interaction. Experiential therapists have been attuned to the affective deficiencies in clients' functioning, and have developed creative methods for facilitating emotional experiencing.

In outlining common principles of change, it must be underscored that this provides a starting point for any attempt to work on psychotherapy integration. If therapists of different theoretical persuasions can acknowledge that these principles of change may be found in the way they work clinically, then the next step would be to examine how these principles are differentially implemented within the clinical context. Thus, within any given case, is there more of an emphasis on increasing awareness about thinking, emotion, or behavior? To what extent is there a focus on awareness of intrapersonal versus interpersonal factors? How much awareness is needed before corrective experiences are called for? These are very real questions that may be fruitfully dealt with by therapists of varying orientations, as they directly address what we actually need to do within the context of a clinical session. Hopefully, we will move toward a point where what we focus on clinically will depend more on the case at hand than our theoretical orientation of origin.

Although interest in working toward psychotherapy integration has gained popularity since the 1980s, it is important to be aware that along with this movement comes the danger of premature attempts at integration. When the Society for the Exploration of Psychotherapy Integration (SEPI) was formed in 1983, the word "exploration" was included in the name to emphasize *the process* of working toward something. I must confess, however, that I often attend SEPI meetings with a conflicting wish and fear. I go with the hope that someone will propose a novel and effective method for integrating the therapies; I also fear that someone will attempt to do so.

My concern is that the psychotherapy integration movement may inadvertently launch a new wave of competitive systems, each vying to become *the* best integrative system available. And while competition has historically served to advance scientific fields, within the realm of psychotherapy, it has tended to result more in proliferation and confusion. Efforts at psychotherapy integration must occur within a collaborative, not competitive context, the goal being to increase our clinical effectiveness rather than further any individual's integrative school of thought. In short, we need to address ourselves to *what* is correct, not *who* is correct.

CONCLUDING COMMENT

In order for change to occur—both in our clients and ourselves as therapists—an understanding and supportive interpersonal context is needed, be it a therapist or colleagues willing to support theoretical openness. An important function of this interpersonal context is to help those interested in change to become more aware of their outmoded methods of functioning, ways that may be undermining what they hope to accomplish. It is within this context that both clients and therapists can become more willing to acknowledge that they inadvertently may be limiting themselves. With this increased awareness, they become better able to consider the possibility of taking risks, so as to try out new ways of thinking, acting, and feeling. These corrective experiences are essential in helping them to update how they understand themselves and others, and ultimately to develop new and hopefully more effective ways of functioning.

Part II
COGNITIVE-BEHAVIORAL ASSESSMENT AND THE THERAPEUTIC CHANGE PROCESS

In the history of clinical psychology, professional involvement in psychotherapy within the U.S. followed psychologists' interest in assessment. It grew out of a need — a need for more therapists during World War II in the 1940s. In cognitive-behavioral assessment, the reverse seems to have been the case. The behavior therapy organization in this country is called the Association for the Advancement of Behavior Therapy, and its primary interest was initially in intervention. Only after it became clear that we could not possibly carry out a clinically sophisticated intervention without an initial assessment, or conduct outcome research without appropriate dependent measures, did we begin to realize that work needed to be done in this area

One of the essential differences between a behavioral and a traditional approach to assessment was described in Mischel's (1968) *Personality and Assessment*. This highly influential work made the point that it was not an individual's motive, drive, or trait that caused the person to behave in a certain way. Instead, argued Mischel, the unit of investigation needed to consist of "what a person *does* in situations rather than on inferences about what attributes he *has* more globally" (Mischel, 1968, p. 10). Mischel's thesis made a most significant impact on the field. But in fairness to others who made similar points before him, they need to be acknowledged as well. For example, the writings of Kurt Lewin, Harry Sack Sullivan, and Julian Rotter all emphasized the important role of the situation as a determinant of behavior. Less well known is the work of Wendell Johnson, especially his book *People in Quandries*, published in 1946. Long before behavioral assessment, or indeed behavior therapy, was even on the horizon, Johnson suggested the following:

> To say that Henry is mean implies that he has some sort of inherent trait, but it tells nothing about what Henry has done. Consequently, it fails to suggest any specific means of improving Henry. If, on the other hand, it is said that Henry snatched Billy's cap and threw it in the bonfire, the situation is rendered somewhat more clear and actually more helpful. You might never eliminate "meanness," but there are fairly definite steps to be taken in order to remove Henry's incentives or opportunities for throwing caps in bonfires. . . .
>
> What the psychiatrist has to do . . . is to get the person to tell him not what he *is* or what he *has*, but what he *does*, and the conditions under which he does it. When he stops talking about what *type* of person he *is*, what his outstanding *traits are*, and what *type* of disorders he *has* — when he stops making these subject-predicate statements, and begins to use actional terms to describe his behavior and its circumstances — both he and the psychiatrist begin to see what specifically may be done in order to change both the behavior and the circumstances. (p. 220)

In 1966, Wallace suggested that the search for an appropriate unit of analysis should be based on an "abilities" view of personality. His thesis was that in conceptualizing personality, it would be helpful if we thought in terms of skills or proficiencies. Just as we would consider assessing the adequacy of a person with regard to a particular role, such as the skills needed to be a competent secretary, so can we construe individuals' personalities in terms of how they deal with various life situations. In a chapter by D'Zurilla and myself, appearing a couple of years later (Goldfried & D'Zurilla, 1969), we picked up on this notion and provided a behavioral conception of "competence." What we meant by competence was the effectiveness with which a individual is able to cope with a problematic life situation, so as to resolve the problematic nature of the situation with a minimal number of negative consequences, and hopefully with positive consequences in other areas of that person's life.

Although behavioral assessment for purposes of case formulation and clinical decision-making received increasing attention in the 1970s, certain events in the 1980s tended to eclipse this aspect of assessment. With the use of disorder-relevant therapy manuals as a means of training clinicians, it appeared as if there was less of a need to conduct an individualized assessment. These manuals, a by-product of clinical trials to determine the efficacy of varying cognitive-behavioral methods for dealing with different clinical problems, contained little in the way of initial assessment prior to intervention. Indeed, the research protocol dictated that therapists should not deviate from the carefully specified manual. Ironically enough, this went counter to the behavioral assessment guidelines described in the 1960s and 1970s, which strongly recommended that clinicians conduct a behavioral analysis so as to tailor their interventions to the particular case. Thus, as therapists have begun to learn cognitive-behavioral procedures by reading these research-based manuals, the issue of assessment for therapeutic planning has tended to fall by the wayside. Fortunately, more recent recognition on the part of practicing clinicians (e.g., Persons, 1989) has raised the consciousness of cognitive-behavior therapists and provided a renewed involvement in clinical assessment.

The first selection in this section, and indeed my first written piece on behavior therapy, describes assessment as a crucial step in the practice of clinical behavior therapy. Written in collaboration with David Pomeranz, it discusses the need to assess the variables associated with the therapeutic change process, and departs from traditional assessment by emphasizing the importance of environmental variables as an important determinant of behavior. In addition, it makes a case to move away from the more radically operant-oriented approach to behavior therapy that began the behavioral movement in the 1960s. In working with adult outpatients, rather than children or hospitalized patients, there is clearly a need to attend to cognitive variables. This selection, consequently, represents part of a trend in the 1960s, where such contributors to the behavioral literature as Bandura, Lazarus, and Mischel argued for the importance of incorporating cognition into behavior therapy. The selection also includes a case illustration in which a cognitive-behavioral formulation of agoraphobia is presented—one that is very much consistent with contemporary thinking in the treatment of this clinical problem.

Chapter 3 deals directly with the distinction between behavioral and more traditional approaches to assessment. Based on an article written with Ronald Kent, it extends the conceptual contributions made by Mischel and others on the behavioral conceptualization of personality, spelling out some of the implications that this conception has when one goes about attempting to actually develop assessment procedures that are consistent with a behavioral orientation. Although the distinction was made in the early 1970s, it is particularly interesting to note that behavioral assessment has since been incorporated into the mainstream of assessment in general. Thus, in an article appearing in the *American Psychologist*, Korchin and Schuldberg (1981) commented on the current status and future direction of clinical assessment, concluding that assessment was still alive and experiencing a renewed sense of vitality. As an illustration of this renewal, they observed a conceptual shift that very much reflected a behavioral influence: more of an emphasis on focal assessment procedures; a greater recognition of the situational determinants of behavior; fewer inferential steps that are taken in the interpretation of test responses; and more attention being paid to a person's evaluation of self and life circumstances.

As behavior therapists began to recognize the relevance of cognition, their interest was naturally drawn to the task of cognitive assessment. A wide variety of procedures have been developed for sampling cognitions, either prior to entering to a situation, during performance itself, or afterward. Most of the initial clinical and research work that has been done in cognitive-behavioral assessment has tended to deal with cognitive products—samples of the individual's thoughts in particular situations. It is only in more recent years that attempts have been made to assess the cognitive processes and structures that may be inferred by these products. In doing so, cognitive-behavior therapy has begun to draw on the work of experimental cognitive psychology. Chapter 4 discusses the role of context in contributing to the semantic meaning individuals attribute to events, and examples are given from the experimental literature as well as from clinical experience. The concept of "schema" is suggested as a way of understanding the potential distortions that may occur when an individual interacts with the environment, by virtue of selective attention, inappropriate classification of events, idiosyncratic storage of information, and/or inaccurate retrieval from memory. A variety of different means by which semantic schemes may be assessed are described.

2

Role of Assessment in Behavior Therapy

Although research in and investigation of behavior therapy proceeded at a rapid pace in the 1960s, one topic that was conspicuously neglected was that of assessment. By assessment we do not solely mean the measurement or other determination of the personality structure of the individual who is the object of some therapeutic endeavor. In using the term assessment, we are referring to the identification and measurement of a broad spectrum of relevant factors that are necessary to ensure the best possible alteration of a particular individual's maladaptive behavior. Indeed, our thesis is that assessment procedures represent a most crucial and significant step in the effective application of behavior therapy.

A significant issue related to the behavior therapist's avoidance of assessment is the traditional conceptualization of personality on which most assessment techniques have been based. The units for understanding human behavior employed by most personality theorists have generally been dispositional in nature. Concepts such as "instincts," "needs," "drives," and "traits" have been the ones most frequently utilized in thinking about personality structure, with these variables having been "assumed to operate as motivational determinants of behavior across varied stimulus situations" (Wallace, 1967, p. 57). This general approach to understanding the determinants of human behavior, namely, emphasizing dynamics, needs, expectations, and underlying motivational forces, has been referred to by Murray (1938) as representing a *centralistic* orientation. We would agree with Wallace, however, who criticizes this approach not only on the grounds that it is conceptually limited, but also that it often leads us into blind alleys in our attempts to predict and change human behavior.

Perhaps the most important reason why behavior therapists originally neglected the area of assessment was their partial or total rejection of the centralistic orientation underlying the available procedures themselves. Operating within the broad framework of learning theory and general experimental research, behavior therapists have not been concerned with conceptualizing personality in any traditional sense. Rejecting the traditional formulations of personality, some behavior therapists have focused entirely on the role of extra-individual factors in the determination of human behavior. They placed great stress on the importance of the stimulus configuration of the environment, and many of the techniques subsumed under the rubric of behavior therapy involve the alteration of the surrounding environment in order to produce change in an individual's behavior. The fact that this emphasis on external determinants resulted in the relative neglect of intra-individual variables is a point we discuss later in the chapter.

BEHAVIOR THERAPY TECHNIQUES AND ASSESSMENT

One of the main reasons for the popularity of the behavior therapy movement in the 1960s is that it offered to the clinician an array of highly specific and seemingly effective techniques. Unfortunately, this led many to view behavior therapy as representing a "new school" of therapy. We would hold that it was neither a school nor was it new. In the first place, it was an eclectic selection of techniques, many of which have been in existence for some time. More important, behavior therapy represented more a general *orientation* to treatment than it did any specific set of techniques. The orientation taken by "behavioral clinicians" was the view that any laws or principles that had been derived from research have possible applications for change in the clinical situation. Basic to this approach was the obvious desire to keep clinical practice firmly based on empirical findings. Although behavior therapy in the clinical setting was most frequently identified with the application of findings from learning studies, the results from experimentation on persuasion, social influence, placebo effect, attitude change, and other topics relevant to the modification of human behavior were equally appropriate (Goldstein, Heller, & Sechrest, 1966).

Several criticisms of the simplistic nature of behavior therapy came from individuals unsympathetic to this orientation (Strupp, 1967; Weitzman, 1967). Of greater significance and concern to us, however, is that criticisms were also leveled by behavior therapists themselves—criticisms that particularly point to the clinical naïveté often reflected in the application of behavior therapy procedures (Davison, 1969; Lazarus, 1965; Meyer & Crisp, 1966). These criticisms apply not so much to the behavior therapy technique per se as they do to the inadequacy of the assessment procedures employed. The two general areas in which this inadequacy is most evident are in (a) the assessment of the most crucial *targets* (behavioral as well as environmental) for modification and (b) the selection of the most appropriate and effective *behavior therapy technique*.

In both case studies and research in behavior therapy, one often has seen gross oversimplification reflected in the conceptualization of the behavior or situation that is seen as being in need of change. For example, the emergence of what appeared to be "symptom substitution" after the application of behavior therapy techniques may be viewed as an instance where the inappropriate target behavior was changed. Modification of maladaptive, anxiety-reducing behavior could very well result in the appearance of another maladaptive response, fairly high in the person's behavior repertoire, which may persist because of its ability to reduce anxiety (Lazarus, 1965). An example of the inappropriate selection of the specific behavior therapy procedure is most dramatically seen in those cases where the client ends up being even more disturbed after the treatment. For example, even though there are instances in which aversive conditioning has proven to be quite successful (Ullmann & Krasner, 1965), there are several cases reported in the literature where it has failed miserably (Beech, 1960; Thorpe & Schmidt, 1963), apparently because it was the inappropriate procedure to use in these particular cases.

It is evident that a more detailed, sophisticated approach to assessment for behavior therapy was needed. The need for clinical assessment to delineate relevant "targets" toward which change should be directed, as well as a means of determining which of the several behavior therapy procedures would be most appropriate and effective, is discussed in the following sections.

Conceptualization of "Targets" for Change

During the 1960s, clinical psychologists began to change their orientation in the study of human behavior. Although once highly centralistic, clinicians and personality theorists alike moved increasingly in the direction of recognizing the significant role of the *concurrent environment* as an influence on human behavior (Kanfer & Saslow, 1965; Rotter, 1960; Sells, 1963; Wallace, 1967). This conceptualization was certainly nothing new; personality theorists spoke about the importance of environmental determinants some years earlier (Lewin, 1939; Murphy, 1947). What was new and exciting, however, is that this conceptualization of human behavior began to receive serious attention by clinicians in their approach to behavior change.

While this increasing emphasis on the role of environmental variables in determining behavior was a welcome one, the exclusion of all inferential concepts and the refusal to consider mediating factors was an untenable orientation that severely limited clinicians in their conceptualizations and therapeutic endeavors. A completely environmentalistic, noninferential orientation to the study of human behavior—which Murray (1938) referred to as the *peripheralistic* approach—does as much violence to the data as does an entirely centralistic orientation. Most behaviorists in the 1960s indeed progressed beyond the simple and naïve approach of conceptualizing behavior merely in terms of overt, molar responses, and developed mediational constructs in terms of which unobservable events can be construed (Hebb, 1960). The application of general principles of behavior to internal, unobservable events resulted in valuable theoretical constructs such as "higher mental processes" (Dollard & Miller, 1950), "symbolic processes" (Mowrer, 1960), "implicit responses" (Staats & Staats, 1963), and "coverants" (Homme, 1965), which enable the theorist and clinician to conceptualize more complex human behavior.

In an intriguing discussion of personality assessment, Wallace (1967) offered what appears to be a compromise between a centralistic and peripheralistic approach in describing an "abilities" conceptualization of personality. In place of the general notion that human behavior can be accounted for by certain learned and innate dispositional characteristics of the individual, complex human behavior may be viewed in the same way that more specific human abilities have been typically conceptualized. Thus, Wallace used the term *response capability* to refer to the extent to which certain responses or behavioral tendencies exist within the person's repertoire. *Response performance*, on the other hand, which refers to the likelihood that the individual will manifest these behavioral tendencies, is determined not only by the extent to which the person is capable of behaving in a given way but also those environmental factors that might tend to elicit and/or reinforce this way of behaving.

In assessing the target behaviors that are in need of change for any given client, it would indeed be simplistic to view behavior as referring to only that which is directly observable. Despite the broadened conceptualization of behavior that became associated with behaviorism in the 1960s, gross oversimplification was often reflected in the selection of target behaviors in case studies and research in behavior therapy. Some behavior therapists failed to recognize that the most appropriate targets for change often involved cognitions as well as overt behaviors. Although we would not deny the fact that thoughts and feelings can sometimes be modified by changing the individual's overt behavior, quite often they should be target behaviors for direct change themselves. Further, although the alteration of consequent events is often effective in eliminating maladaptive behavior, the importance of changes in the situational antecedents should not be overlooked.

We would agree with Szasz (1961) that the general goal of therapy should be the elimination of the individual's problems in living. Clearly, these problems in living may be primarily a function of individuals' behavioral abilities or deficits, their current environmental situation, but more likely some combination of the two (cf. Wallace, 1967). Consequently, in the selection of the "target" to be the focus of change, the clinician should choose from: (a) the relevant antecedent, situational events that may have elicited the maladaptive behavior; (b) the cognitive mediational responses and cues which, because of the individual's previous learning experiences, have become associated with these situational events; (c) the observable, maladaptive behavior itself; and (d) the consequent changes in the environmental situation, including the reactions of others. The decision as to which aspect of this environmental-mediational-behavioral complex is most relevant in any case should be determined by which, if effectively changed, is most likely to alter the client's maladaptive behavior. An illustration of the use of this paradigm in a case study is presented later in the chapter.

Selection of Appropriate Behavior Therapy Procedures

In addition to using assessment procedures to determine the target for change, assessment is essential in the selection of the therapeutic technique most appropriate for any given case. Unlike many therapists of other orientations, behaviorally-oriented clinicians find themselves faced with the task of having to choose from a wide range of possible procedures, each of which seems to have had some success clinically (Bandura, 1961; Goldstein et al., 1966; Ullmann & Krasner, 1965). The behavior therapist must decide whether the most appropriate approach to take with any given client should involve such techniques as desensitization, assertion training, role-playing techniques, modeling procedures, or any one of a variety of other approaches. The selection of any given procedure may be in part a function of the target behavior or situational determinant in need of modification. With further investigation of each of the therapeutic procedures, however, it has become clear that other variables may play a significant role as well.

In order to determine which would be the most appropriate therapeutic procedure to employ in any given case, we need to explore the specific variables related to effective application of each of the several behavior therapy procedures. As an example, let us take the use of modeling procedures, since relevant empirical data exist in the use of this procedure. Under what conditions would modeling be an effective procedure to employ clinically? To begin with, research findings by Bandura and his associates (Bandura, 1965; Bandura & Walters, 1963) indicate that modeling is particularly relevant in those instances where, due to inadequate social learning, certain desired behavior patterns are low in the individual's repertoire. Modeling procedures have additionally proven to be relevant in those instances where avoidance responses need to be eliminated (Bandura, Grusec, & Menlove, 1967).

Apart from delineating these particular target behaviors, however, any assessment procedure would also have to focus on *other* client and environmental variables relevant to the effective application of modeling. We have already spoken of the importance of assessing environmental and client variables in determining the relevant targets for change. Our interest in these variables now lies in making a decision as to whether or not our therapeutic procedure is the most appropriate one to use in this particular situation. In the case of modeling procedures, the assessment would have to provide information about such client characteristics as arousal level, self-esteem, and degree of dependency, as well as data on the nature of the concurrent environmental situation, such as the availability of the appropriate models and the likelihood of the client's behavior being followed by positive consequences (cf. Bandura, 1965; Goldstein et al., 1966).

The issues that have been discussed above regarding the importance of assessment for behavior therapy may perhaps be brought into a clearer focus by the use of an illustrative case.

Illustrative Clinical Case

Consider the hypothetical case of a 50-year-old agoraphobic man who entered therapy because he has difficulty leaving his house. The situation has reached the point where merely contemplating getting out of bed results in such anxiety that most of his time is spent in a prone position, requiring that he be constantly looked after by his wife. Further questioning reveals that his most salient fear is having a heart attack, which he states is the reason for remaining at home and in bed. Upon carrying the assessment further—this time evaluating the nature of his current life situation—it is found that this man has recently been promoted in his job to a position where he now has the responsibility for supervising a large staff. Prior to this promotion, he led a fairly normal life and his fears of having a heart attack were nonexistent.

Other assessment procedures reveal that the client has always had the tendency to become anxious in unfamiliar situations, and he is the type of person who would prefer to have other people look after and care for him. Additionally, questioning his wife reveals that she does not find the current situation entirely noxious; rather, she feels important and needed now that she has to care for her husband, and she lavishes much attention and affection on him in his incapacitated state.

Prior to the delineation of the appropriate target for change, the clinician must conceptualize the case more systematically. As we have noted above, a formulation should focus on: (a) the relevant environmental antecedents, (b) the significant mediational responses and cues, (c) the observable maladaptive behavior itself, and (d) the consequent environmental changes.

Using this paradigm, a formulation of this case might be as follows: the change in this individual's work situation elicited a number of mediating (cognitive) responses (e.g., this is a situation requiring direction and supervision of others, judgments must be made about other people's performance, inadequate work of others reflects negatively on a supervisor, etc.). Because of this particular individual's previous learning experiences, these cognitions, associated with a change in job status, elicit anxiety. Among the many manifestations of this anxiety reaction is an increase in heart rate. Because of the client's mislabeling of this state of increased arousal, i.e., he associates the increased activity of the heart in a man of his age and position with the possibility of having a heart attack, he becomes concerned with thoughts that this might be happening to him. These thoughts serve as mediating responses that tend to elicit additional anxiety, thus adding to his distressed condition. Remaining at home and confined to bed, which belong to a class of behaviors relatively high in his behavioral repertoire, serve as successful avoidance responses that keep him out of the situation initially eliciting the anxiety; it is also appropriate behavior for a person who might be having a heart attack. His behavior results in attention and care from his wife, providing additional reinforcement for the maladaptive behavior.

Following the translation of the data into conceptual terms, the clinician is then faced with the task of selecting the most relevant target for change. The most salient target in this case — the *observable, maladaptive behavior* of staying at home and remaining in bed — does not appear to be the most appropriate for direct modification. We have conceptualized this behavior as an avoidance response, where the stimuli eliciting the anxiety continue to be present. The direct alteration of this overt behavior without any change in the mediating anxiety could very well result in the manifestation of other avoidance responses lower in the client's repertoire. In considering possible modifications in the *current life situation*, we also encounter difficulties. Although a change in the situation that was *antecedent* to the appearance of this maladaptive behavior — his promotion at work — might successfully eliminate the problem, it would also result in a financial and status loss for this individual; the focus on other targets that would eliminate the problem and yet avoid these other negative consequences would be preferable. Dealing with the *consequent* aspect of the client's current life situation—the attention he is receiving from his wife—would only be focusing on the additional reinforcers and not on the stimuli that are concurrently eliciting the behavioral avoidance.

Having considered the observable maladaptive behavior and the current life situation as possible areas for modification, we would now turn to the *mediational responses*. The client's distorted labeling of the physiological cues that were a concomitant of the anxiety reaction seems to be of secondary importance. Antecedent to this inappropriate labeling is the anxiety elicited by those situations requiring him to supervise and make decisions about others. It is his fear of functioning in this type of situation that seems to have resulted in a chain of internal and external maladaptive response. It, therefore, appears that the crucial area toward which most of the therapeutic endeavors should be directed would be the client's anxiety regarding decision-making processes in the supervision of others.

Following the selection of the most crucial target for change, some decision must be made in the choice of the most appropriate treatment procedure; it is here where assessment is most inadequate. The assessment of the target makes the task of selecting the appropriate therapeutic procedure less difficult, although certainly not clear-cut. Indeed, what we often find is that the assessment enables us *to eliminate* certain therapeutic techniques more than it does to indicate which would be most appropriate. In the case of our hypothetical client, the determination of whether or not to employ desensitization, modeling techniques, cognitive restructuring, implosive therapy, or perhaps assertion training in the reduction of his anxiety regarding decision-making, cannot easily be made on the basis of any existing assessment information. Although it may well be that one particular approach to anxiety-reduction would be most effective with this client in his particular life situation, we can only speculate about the variables (e.g., imaginal ability, level of anxiety, ability to relax, suggestibility, the reactions of others, etc.) pertinent to the successful application of the above-mentioned techniques.

Although it may be possible to use clinical intuition and experience as an aid in determining what seems to be the most appropriate behavior therapy technique, the typical clinical procedure typically involves selecting a few seemingly relevant techniques and then trying each in turn until one hopefully proves effective. A better strategy would be the determination of those predictive or assessment variables needed in the selection of the most effective treatment in any given case. Such a goal can best be achieved by means of systematic research efforts directed toward discovering these individual and environmental variables. To quote Paul (1967), the relevant research questions to be asked are: "*What* treatment, by *whom*, is most effective for *this* individual with *that* specific problem, and under *which* set of circumstances?" (p. 111). It is toward the goal of answering these questions that the future study of assessment for behavior therapy should be directed.

SUMMARY

The introduction of a broad range of behavior therapy techniques has brought into focus several questions and issues of concern to clinicians and researchers. The particular problem discussed in this chapter has been the need for a formulation of relevant assessment strategies. Some of the possible reasons for the original lack of attention given to assessment by behavior therapists have been presented, followed by a conceptualization of the role of assessment in this approach to treatment. This formulation outlined two general goals toward which assessment should be directed: the delineation of the most relevant "targets" for change and the selection of the most appropriate behavior therapy procedure. A hypothetical case and its formulation was presented to illustrate these proposals, and some directions for future study were noted.

3

Traditional versus Behavioral Personality Assessment

Because the successful implementation of behavior therapy techniques depends directly upon an adequate assessment of the specific targets in need of change and those variables maintaining them, this approach to treatment also stimulated a renewed interest in clinical assessment (Goldfried & Pomeranz, 1968; Kanfer & Saslow, 1969; Mischel, 1968; Peterson, 1968). Greenspoon and Gersten (1967) noted the importance of clinical assessment for the effective application of behavior therapy procedures, and argued for the possible utility of currently available tests of personality. Close examination reveals, however, that there are certain basic assumptions associated with traditional personality tests that make this approach to assessment less appropriate from a behavioral viewpoint. Just as the behavioral framework has been used to generate new therapeutic procedures, it would seem advantageous to use this orientation for the construction of new assessment techniques as well.

Before proceeding further, we would like to note briefly what we mean by "traditional" and "behavioral" approaches to assessment. Although the ultimate goal of both procedures may be essentially the same (e.g., the prediction of human behavior), the general approach that has been employed in the pursuit of this goal has differed. The traditional approach to personality assessment has been directed primarily toward an understanding of the individual's underlying personality characteristics or traits as a means of predicting behavior. This general approach to assessment is reflected in most personality tests — both projective techniques (Rorschach, Thematic Apperception Test, Draw-A-Person, etc.) as well as objective personality inventories (Minnesota Multiphasic Personality Inventory [MMPI], California Psychological Inventory, etc.). The behavioral approach to personality assessment, by contrast, involves more of a direct measurement of the individual's response to various life situations. The techniques associated with behavioral assessment include the observation of individuals in naturalistic situations, the creation of an experimental analogue of real-life situations via role playing, and the utilization of the individual's self-reported responses to given situations.

These two general approaches to personality assessment may be differentiated on a pragmatic level as well. In the case of the traditional procedures, the focus has been on the accuracy with which they might be used to predict behavior, with relatively little emphasis being placed on their utility for selecting therapeutic procedures (cf. Meehl, 1960). The therapeutic approach employed in any given case is usually more a function of the therapist's particular orientation than it is of psychological test findings (Goldfried & Pomeranz, 1968; London, 1964). By contrast, the interest in behavioral assessment has been generated by its utility for providing the information essential to the selection and implementation of appropriate behavior therapy procedures. Some of the possible reasons underlying the differential clinical utility of the two approaches have been noted in Chapter 2 and are not dealt with here. Instead, the primary point of comparison on which we focus involves those assumptions underlying each approach, as well as the potential use each has for accurately predicting human behavior.

Although traditional personality tests and behavioral tests share many of the same methodological assumptions (e.g., reliability of scoring, adequacy of standardization) the primary purpose of this chapter is to compare the *differing* assumptions involved in these two approaches. The basic conception of personality and those assumptions associated with the selection of test items and the interpretation of test responses are first described and evaluated for both traditional and behavioral approaches to assessment, after which a comparison is drawn between these two approaches for predicting human behavior.

ASSUMPTIONS INVOLVED IN THE TRADITIONAL APPROACH TO ASSESSMENT

Conception of Personality

Most of our personality tests are based on a common conceptualization of human functioning, and have been directed toward obtaining information relevant to the underlying "personality structure" of the individual. Depending upon one's specific theoretical orientation, these inferred characteristics may consist of "motives," "needs," "drives," "defenses," "traits," or other similar psychodynamic constructs. For the most part, the various psychodynamic or trait theories are based on the notion of psychic determinism, whereby a person's actions are assumed to be motivated by certain underlying dynamics. According to this conception of personality, the most appropriate way in which to predict human behavior should be based on a thorough assessment of those inferred characteristics of which the overt actions are believed to be a function.

Basic to the traditional conception of personality functioning is the assumption that consistencies in behavior (i.e., traits) exist independent of situational variations. Data from several studies, however, have failed to support this assumption. The effect of varying stimulus conditions on behavior has been demonstrated by Hartshorne and May's (1928) classic study on honesty, in which children were provided with opportunities to cheat, lie, and steal in a diversity of settings (e.g., home, party games, athletics). Hartshorne and May found a lack of a generalized code of morals, and concluded that "as we progressively change the situation we progressively lower the correlations between the tests [p. 384]." Endler and Hunt (1966, 1969) have similarly demonstrated the importance of situational effects in their S-R Inventory of Anxiousness, where they found that the interactions between situations and subjects contributed more to the total variance than did the variance associated with individual differences alone. On the basis of both questionnaire data and direct observations, Moos (1969) similarly found a substantial proportion of the variance resulting from Subject X Setting interactions. Although Mischel and Ebbesen (1970) have reported individual differences among children in the ability to delay gratification, it was possible to substantially modify the period of delay by creating variations in the particular situation. Mischel (1968) has reviewed a number of other studies dealing with this issue, the results of which have failed to confirm the conception of human functioning that does not take into account the importance of environmental influences on behavior.

Selection of Test Items

An important consequence of the view that consistencies in behavior exist independent of situational variables has been the fact that relatively little emphasis has been placed on how to select the pool of stimulus items for traditional tests of personality (Loevinger, 1957). Although test constructors often employ rigorous selection procedures to obtain a final set of items, the procedures for defining the original pool are rarely discussed. This original item pool is obviously not determined on a random basis, but is presumably related to the test constructor's assumptions regarding the nature of the personality variables in question.

Loevinger (1957) and Jessor and Hammond (1957) have criticized this poorly defined approach to selecting the initial set of items, and suggested instead the use of a specific theoretical orientation as an alternate guide in selecting the item pool. In using personality theory to select these items, one assumes that the theory in question has some "validity." Although certain constructs associated with specific theoretical orientations have received some research support, there does not appear to be any one personality theory which, as yet, has achieved adequate enough empirical confirmation to justify such an approach to item selection.

Interpretation of Test Responses

While variations in the stimulus aspects of the test situation have been considered to be relatively unimportant, the interpretation of responses has been the subject of extensive and detailed consideration. The interpretive significance of any particular test response may be determined by either *intuitive* or *empirical* means (Hase & Goldberg, 1967; Loevinger, 1957). The intuitive approach may be based on an informal rationale with few explicit theoretical assumptions, or may involve more formal deductions from theory. In using the empirical approach, on the other hand, the interpretive significance of test responses is derived solely from the empirically established relationship between test and external criteria.

Even in those instances where the intuitive approach is used initially to specify the interpretive significance of various signs, empirical checks on the accuracy of those interpretations are clearly needed. However, logical or theoretical assumptions underlying the meaning of test signs are often so firmly held that failure to obtain empirical confirmation often has little effect on changing clinicians' interpretations. Thus, despite evidence indicating that Hutt and Briskin's (1960) proposed interpretation of various signs lacks empirical confirmation (Goldfried & Ingling, 1964), the revised edition of the manual (Hutt, 1968) continued to recommend the use of invalid interpretations.

The tendency for clinicians to retain certain interpretive hypotheses about test scores is directly illustrated in a study by Chapman and Chapman (1969), where they asked experienced psychodiagnosticians to determine which of several Rorschach signs reflected male homosexuality. The signs presented to the clinicians were selected from Wheeler's (1949) initial list of 20 possible Rorschach indicators of homosexuality, only some of which have held up under empirical test. The results indicated that clinicians tended to select those signs that they believed to be most indicative of male homosexuality on a rational-intuitive basis (e.g., "buttocks") — despite the fact that research findings failed to confirm the empirical validity of these signs — and almost never selected those indices that were, in fact, empirically valid. As noted by the authors, these "illusory correlations" between sign and inferred characteristics are likely to be a source of considerable error in predicting criterion behaviors.

Although such illusory correlations are only a problem for intuitively derived tests, other potential sources of error exist with empirically derived measures. For example, despite the fact that the clinical scales on the MMPI were originally derived to assist in diagnostic classification, the test has been used for more complex decisions (Dahlstrom & Welsh, 1960). Rather than simply using an MMPI protocol to determine diagnostic category, the clinician more typically carries out a profile analysis, in which both the absolute and relative scores on the various scales are used to construct a personality description. Any such interpretation must assume a high correspondence between the diagnostic categories associated with the scales and the inferred personality traits. Such an assumption, however, has failed to receive empirical support, in that considerable overlap in behavioral characteristics has been found to exist among the various diagnostic classifications (Mischel, 1968; Zigler & Phillips, 1961).

Another assumption basic to the interpretation of test responses is that the protocol provides a sufficient sampling of the individual's personality characteristics (MacFarlane & Tuddenham, 1951; Murstein, 1961). In the case of a projective techniques, Murstein acknowledged that since this "sampling" is determined by the subject's own response to the test situation — which differs from individual to individual — one cannot always be certain that sufficient data have, in fact, been obtained. In the case of objective tests, guidelines for determining the adequacy of the sample are virtually nonexistent, with the exception of Loevinger's (1957) suggestion that theory serve as the background for test construction.

ASSUMPTIONS INVOLVED IN THE BEHAVIORAL APPROACH TO ASSESSMENT

Conception of Personality

In contrast to the psychodynamic orientation, which focuses on the characteristics an individual "has," the behavioral view of human functioning places greater emphasis on what a person "does" in various situations (Mischel, 1968). That is, rather than hypothesizing certain underlying constructs (e.g., "instincts" or "needs") that are believed to function as motivational determinants of behavior, the basic unit for consideration involves the individual's response to specific aspects of his environment. Human behavior is viewed as being determined not only by the person's previous social learning history but also by current environmental antecedents and/or consequences of the behavior in question.

As noted in Chapter 2, the behavioral orientation to personality is well represented by Wallace's (1967) "abilities" conception. Wallace used the concept *response capability* as referring to the individual's behavioral repertoire or potential, which is determined primarily by earlier learning experiences. This closely parallels what is typically referred to when one speaks of an acquired skill, such as the ability to drive a car, ride a bicycle, or other learned proficiencies. The likelihood that an individual will actually *perform* in a given way, however, will depend on the extent to which certain situational factors elicit and/or reinforce this particular response. From this point of view, then, personality may be construed as an intervening variable that is defined according to the likelihood of an individual manifesting certain behavioral tendencies in the variety of situations that comprise his or her day-to-day living.

As noted in conjunction with our discussion of the traditional conception of personality, the available research evidence does, in fact, indicate that the likelihood of individual's responding in a certain way depends not only on their own response capability but also on the nature of the situation as well (cf. Endler & Hunt, 1966, 1969; Hartshorne & May, 1928; Mischel & Ebbesen, 1970; Moos, 1969). After reviewing the experimental literature regarding the consistency of personality variables, Mischel (1968) has concluded that "behaviors which are often construed as stable personality trait indicators actually are highly specific and depend on the details of the evoking situations and the response mode employed to measure them [p. 37]."

Selection of Test Items

Consistent with a conception of personality that emphasizes the individual's specific response to specific situations, a crucial assumption of behavioral tests is that stimulus situations are adequately represented. Adequate representation of situations requires not only careful simulation during the measurement process (e.g., video depictions, written descriptions) but also rigorous definition of the appropriate pool of situations. For example, in surveying fear behavior (Geer, 1965; Wolpe & Lang, 1964), it is necessary to obtain measures of fear in situations that sample, in a representative manner, the population of potentially anxiety-producing situations. In selecting the stimulus items, then, the concept of content validity, as it has been traditionally applied to proficiency tests, becomes highly relevant for behavioral assessment.

Goldfried and D'Zurilla (1969) have followed this line of thinking and developed a "behavioral analytic" method for test construction. For example, Goldfried and D'Zurilla have applied the behavioral analytic model in the study of college freshman effectiveness by identifying those responses that are differentially rewarded by significant individuals in situations that define the college environment. The initial step in selecting a pool of test items consists of a "situational analysis," in order to obtain a sample of problematic situations that were likely to be encountered by freshmen during their first semester. The situational analysis was accomplished by means of written daily records of problematic situations obtained from freshmen themselves, as well as through interviews with staff members having frequent contact with freshmen. The large pool of situations resulting from these procedures was then presented to a new sample of freshmen during the second semester, who were asked to indicate which of these situations they had ever encountered. Only those instances that had a high likelihood of occurrence were retained in the item pool. The following is an example of one such situation (Goldfried & D'Zurilla, 1969):

> A lengthy composition is due in your English class this Friday. It was assigned a week before and is on a rather difficult topic, which you really don't understand.
> On Wednesday afternoon when you sit down to work, you find that you have absolutely no idea about what to include in the paper. You realize, however, that you must start writing the composition soon in order to have it in on time.

This approach to the selection of an item pool carries with it the assumption that the informants have provided an accurate account of the problematic situations associated with the college environment, as well as the assumption that the particular situations selected will continue to have a high probability of occurrence over the period of time during which the assessment is to take place. These assumptions are capable of direct empirical confirmation by utilizing a different group of informants, and by surveying the frequency of occurrence of these situations at a later point in time.

Interpretation of Test Responses

In discussing the assumptions underlying the interpretation of behavioral tests, we may note the basic distinction drawn by Goodenough (1949) between the "sign" and the "sample" approaches to interpreting test responses. The sign approach assumes that the response may best be construed as an indirect manifestation of some underlying personality characteristic. The sample approach, on the other hand, assumes that the test behavior constitutes a subset of the actual behaviors of interest. Whereas traditional personality tests have typically taken the sign approach to interpretation, behavioral procedures approach test interpretation with the sample orientation.

The assumption that behavioral test responses constitute a sample of certain response tendencies is closely tied to the assumption that the test items themselves consist of a representative sample of situations relevant to the behaviors of interest. In the assessment of assertiveness toward authority, for example, a sampling interpretation of the individual's test responses would rest on the assumption that the test items represent an adequate sample of interpersonal situations involving authority figures.

Another issue related to the interpretation of test behavior as a sample of criterion behavior is that of the *method* employed for the expression of the response. The ideal approach to response expression would constitute the individual's actual response in a real-life situation, in that this represents the most direct approach to behavioral sampling. Within certain settings, such as hospitals and classrooms, this approach can be readily implemented. Unless these observations are unobtrusive, the assumption that the behavior remains unaffected by the assessment procedures may turn out to be faulty. For example, a study by Patterson and Harris (1968) suggests that such considerations as deciding to have an outside observer, rather than the mother herself, make observations of her child's behavior in the home may produce differences in the data obtained. Moos (1968) similarly found a tendency for hospitalized patients to respond differently when they were aware that their behavior was being observed.

In instances where unobtrusive direct observation procedures are not feasible, other approaches to response expression must be employed. A potentially useful alternative consists of role-playing procedures, where individuals are required to act out their response as if they were actually in the situation in question. The available research on the use of role playing for assessment offers some support for the assumption that the role-played response parallels the behavior in the real-life setting. For example, in an attempt to predict competent behavior under conditions of interpersonal stress, Stanton and Litwak (1955) found that subjects' responses to role-playing situations involving such stress correlated .82 with independent ratings by informants who were familiar with the subjects' behavior in this type of situation. Further support for the value of role playing as an assessment procedure comes from the work of Weiss (1968) on the prediction of "reinforcing skill" in interpersonal situations. This assessment technique consists of placing subjects in a role-playing situation where they are asked to listen to a speaker and do whatever they can to "maintain rapport" with this individual. The frequency of subjects' reinforcing behaviors as recorded in the role-playing assessment has been found to be predictive of peer ratings for social behavior (e.g., "fun at a party"), and of independent ratings of the competence and reinforcing skill among therapists.

Still another approach in assessing an individual's response is through self-reports of behavior. The assumption associated with the use of self-report is that individuals can accurately observe and communicate their reactions to certain situations. The most extensive use of self-report procedures has been in conjunction with the assessment of anxiety. In the use of fear survey schedules, for example, a list of potentially frightening objects (e.g., blood, spiders) and situations (e.g., being criticized, being alone) is presented to individuals, who must indicate the extent to which they subjectively find each of these to be frightening. Findings by Geer (1965) indicate that subjects' responses to specific items on the fear survey schedule (i.e., dogs, rats) were predictive of their fear reaction when placed in an actual situation where they had to approach these objects. Paul's (1966) successful use of the S-R Inventory of Anxiousness to predict anxiety in a public speaking situation ($r = .50$ and $.72$ for two separate samples) similarly adds credibility to the assumption that verbal self-prediction bears a good correspondence to behavior in real-life situations.

The use of direct observation, role playing, or self-report procedures for behavioral assessment is based on the assumption that the particular method selected contributes little variance to the responses that are sampled. Although it is possible that the results obtained by using each of these different methods will differ, there currently exists no research evidence bearing on this question. Using Campbell and Fiske's (1959) suggested approach to studying method variance, however, the degree of correspondence among responses obtained through these different procedures can readily be subjected to direct empirical test.

In addition to the question of the particular method employed in the assessment procedures, there is also the issue of how to *categorize* or *score* this response. Rather than attempting to develop scoring keys based on either intuitive or empirical grounds, the behavioral approach to assessment utilizes information about the actual criterion behaviors—that is, those behaviors that are the target of the prediction. In the case of the S-R Inventory of Anxiousness (Endler & Hunt, 1966, 1969), for example, 14 "modes of response" were selected to assess the individual's "anxiety" reaction to any given situation. These several modes of response (e.g., heart beating faster, getting an uneasy feeling, wanting to avoid a situation, perspiring) were chosen to represent the multidimensional character that has been found to typify the actual fear response (cf. Lang, 1968).

In their description of the behavioral analytic approach to assessing competence, Goldfried and D'Zurilla (1969) have suggested guidelines for conducting a criterion analysis to be used in establishing standards for scoring behavioral measures. This behaviorally oriented criterion analysis consists of (*a*) a *situational analysis*, in which the relevant environmental events are sampled: (*b*) a *response enumeration*, where a pool of responses for each of these several situations is obtained; and (*c*) the *response evaluation*, which entails the categorization of each potential course of action in a situation according to its degree of effectiveness. So as to parallel the "actual" effectiveness of these several behaviors in the real-life setting, it is recommended that the judgments of effectiveness be made by "significant others"—that is, individuals who are respected by those people toward whom the assessment is being directed, and who have the role of labeling behavior as being effective or ineffective in that particular environment.

The basic assumption underlying this approach to establishing scoring criteria is that there exist common standards or behavioral norms for effectiveness within the particular life setting in question, and that these standards are relatively stable over the period of time during which the assessment is to take place. In light of the rapidly changing value system associated with many aspects of our society, this assumption may prove to be faulty in the assessment of certain behaviors (e.g., students' interactions with authority). It should be emphasized, however, that failure to confirm empirically the existence of a stable set of behavioral norms would have implications not only for the establishment of scoring criteria but also for the selection of criterion behaviors against which any validation could take place. How-

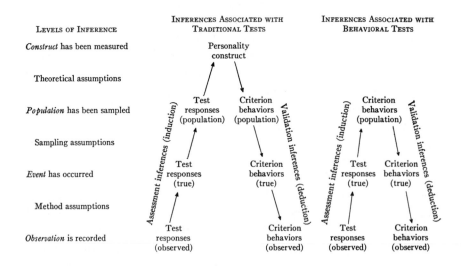

                    INFERENCES ASSOCIATED WITH   INFERENCES ASSOCIATED WITH
  LEVELS OF INFERENCE   TRADITIONAL TESTS   BEHAVIORAL TESTS

FIGURE 3.1

ever, this would pose a problem for any attempt at predicting human behavior, whether it be behavioral or traditional.

COMPARISON OF TRADITIONAL AND BEHAVIORAL ASSESSMENT

At this point, a more direct comparison may be drawn between traditional and behavioral approaches to assessment, taking into account the levels of inference associated with each, and the available data on comparative predictive ability.

Comparative Levels of Inference

In order to compare more systematically the nature of the assumptions involved in traditional and behavioral assessment, the inferences associated with the prediction of behavior from each of these approaches have been depicted graphically in Figure 3.1. The arrows in the figure pointing upward refer to those assessment inferences or in-

ductions associated with the interpretation of the test scores themselves, whereas the arrows pointing downward reflect validation inferences—that is, deductions from the interpretation of the test that are
associated with the prediction of the criterion. The three levels of inference associated with both the induction and deduction include: (*a*)
Those inferences that allow one to conclude that the *recorded observation* accurately reflects the occurrence of some specific *event*,
namely, the "true" test response, or the "true" criterion behavior. This
is clearly the most basic of all inferences and carries with it such assumptions as the reliability with which the test response and criterion
behavior is recorded and scored, as well as the absence of variance
that might be attributed to the specific method employed in assessing
the event in question (cf. Campbell & Fiske, 1959). (*b*) The second
level of inference, in which one concludes that the event being measured is a sample of some *larger population*, is based on the assumption that the responses obtained by the test—or the criterion behaviors
selected for observation—are representative of the relevant aspects of
the entire population of true responses (or criterion behaviors) in
question. (*c*) Following the assumption that the population of responses has been adequately sampled, it may additionally be inferred
that the test performance has been indicative of some unobservable
construct, and in turn, that this construct may be reflected by certain
criterion behaviors. This third level of inference requires theoretical
assumptions that describe the relation between the construct in question, and both the population of responses and the population of criterion behaviors.

Using this schematic outline of levels of inference, we may compare the prediction process from two approaches to assessment. As an
example, consider the prediction of anxiety in relationships with
same-sex peers, first from the traditional point of view and then from
a behavioral approach.

Using a traditional test of personality, the most basic of all assumptions would be that the relevant test responses as observed (e.g.,
presence of inanimate movement on the Rorschach or high social in-
troversion on the MMPI) are only negligibly affected by scoring error
or any artifacts associated with the measurement process itself. These
"true" test responses, in turn, are assumed to constitute an adequate
sample of some hypothetical population of potential anxiety-related
test responses that the particular examinee might give if, for example,

the measure were administered at another time or the length of the test had been extended. Once the adequacy of this sample has been assumed, additional assumptions are required to relate this population of signs to an underlying personality construct believed to be related to anxiety in same-sex peer relations. The construct selected would vary from theory to theory, and might include such inferred characteristics as basic insecurity, conflicts over underlying homosexual tendencies, incongruence between self- and ideal-concept, or other similarly hypothesized variables. In using this information deductively to predict behavior, additional theoretical assumptions are required to relate the inferred personality construct to a population of criterion behaviors that might reflect various anxiety-laden interactions with same-sex peers. Depending upon the particular theory of personality employed at this stage of the prediction process, the behavioral definition is apt to vary. From this hypothetical population of behaviors, specific behavioral interactions are then sampled (e.g., conversational ability in specific social situations), and procedures for measuring these criterion behaviors are selected (e.g., direct observation, peer ratings).

A behavioral test to predict anxiety in same-sex peer relationships, by contrast, would consist of placing the individual in a representative sample of situations requiring peer contact and eliciting his/her response. Inasmuch as this procedure might take any one of several forms (e.g., direct observations in actual situations, role-playing, self-report), it is assumed that the individual's "true" response contributes more variance than does the particular method selected. The next level of inference is based on the assumption that the elicited responses have provided an adequate sample of potential criterion behaviors that define anxiety in such relationships. In contrast with the traditional approaches to personality assessment, behavioral assessment views the responses given as samples of the criterion behaviors themselves. Further, these behaviors are derived directly from an empirically defined criterion analysis (e.g., sampling situations involving interactions with peers), thereby eliminating the need for either the inductive or deductive use of theoretical assumptions. Once these criterion behaviors to be used for the validation have been specified, essentially the same psychometric procedures employed by traditional personality measures would be used in testing for criterion-related validity.

This comparison between the two approaches to prediction, in fact, is oversimplified. Rarely would a traditional diagnostician predict to a criterion measure, such as anxiety in relations with members of the same sex, on the basis of one type of test response and the inference from one personality construct. Rather, several types of responses, elicited by a battery of different tests, would be evaluated, and several personality constructs inferred. Then, as a further inference involving additional theoretical assumptions, these constructs would be interrelated to provide a dynamic picture of the individual's personality functioning. This attempt to develop a "theory of a person" (cf. Sundberg & Tyler, 1962) involves inferences most removed from the data and most dependent upon the clinician's theoretical orientation and clinical experience.

Even in the more simplified form in which we have presented it, the comparison underlines a crucial difference in the construction of traditional and behavioral tests. To recapitulate, traditional personality tests have developed methods for eliciting behaviors that may serve as signs of underlying personality variables. The responses elicited by the tests serve as a basis for theoretical inferences regarding basic personality functioning, which is then related to criterion measures. By contrast, behavioral tests, such as those following the behavioral analytic model (Goldfried & D'Zurilla, 1969) may be developed by working backward from criterion measures. That is, a sampling of the criterion situation and behaviors is obtained first, after which an attempt is made to develop efficient measurement procedures for assessing these behavior-environment interactions.

Comparative Predictive Ability

It is interesting to note that because of its greater predictive potential, there has been a general leaning over the years toward more direct, criterion-related measures within the realm of traditional personality testing. In conjunction with a review of the prognostic use of various personality measures, for example, Fulkerson and Barry (1961) have concluded that of all the possible ways to predict behavior, the most accurate predictor remains the individual's previous behavior in similar situations.

After reviewing the research on the TAT, Murstein (1963) concluded that certain aspects of the subject's response to the testing situation itself may prove to be potentially useful in predicting overt behavior in the criterion situation. As he noted, however, these responses

> are not really part of the stories, but represent miniature bits of overt behavior similar to the criterion overt behavior. It is small wonder, therefore, that caustic comments in the telling of a TAT story are related to overt aggression. (pp. 318-319)

In a similar vein, Kagan (1956), rather than utilizing theoretical constructs to improve the relationship between TAT scores and overt aggression, was successful in improving predictive ability by using stimulus materials that more accurately sampled the actual criterion situation (rather than the typical ambiguous stimuli), and scored the protocols for only those aspects of aggression (e.g., tendency to fight) that were of interest in the criterion situation.

In the case of the Rorschach, the procedure that most closely approximates scoring and interpreting test responses as a sample of overt behavior has been developed by Friedman (1953). Using Werner's (1948) description of perceptual and cognitive development, Friedman has described a procedure for using each response as a sample of perceptual behavior. In comparison to many of the other approaches to scoring the Rorschach, Friedman's approach stays much closer to the data and involves considerably fewer assumptions and—perhaps as a result of this—has consistently resulted in favorable empirical validation (Goldfried, Stricker, & Weiner, 1971).

In addition to these indirect findings regarding the predictive potential of behavioral assessment, there have been some studies in which a direct comparison was made between the predictive ability of traditional and behavioral assessment procedures. For example, in conjunction with a larger study on the effectiveness of systematic desensitization as a procedure for reducing anxiety in a public speaking situation, Paul (1966) administered a variety of personality measures prior to treatment (Institute for Personality and Ability testing [IPAT] Anxiety Scale, Bendig's Emotionality Scale, Bendig's Extraversion-Introversion Scale, Anxiety Differential, and the S-R Inventory of Anxiousness). Using as a criterion the subjects' personal report of confidence when in a public speaking situation, Paul found that the correlations obtained with the S-R Inventory of Anxiousness item involving public speaking exceeded by far the correlations found with the more traditional tests. Thus, with data from two separate samples, the average correlation obtained between criterion and the S-R Inventory was .61, in comparison to correlations of .15 for IPAT anxiety, of -.24 for extraversion-introversion, .07 for emotionality, and .29 for the Anxiety Differential.

Wallace and Sechrest (1963) conducted a study in which they compared the predictive accuracy of several projective techniques with the subjects' own self-ratings in the assessment of achievement, hostility, somatic concern, and religious concern. The results of the study indicated that whereas the correlations between criterion (peer ratings on each of the variables) and self-ratings on these dimensions averaged .57, the average correlations for the other tests were .05 for the Rorschach, .08 for the TAT, and .14 for Rotter's Incomplete Sentences Blank.

The results of a study reported by Carroll (1952) similarly found simple self-ratings yielded higher correlations than did scores on the Guilford-Martin Personnel Inventory. In an analysis of method variance via a multi-trait multi-method correlation matrix, Campbell and Fiske (1959) have noted that Carroll's findings also suggest that the self-ratings appeared to be less confounded by method variance.

Using the item pool of the California Psychological Inventory, Hase and Goldberg (1967) compared the predictive power of scales constructed by various means (e.g., theoretical, empirical, factor analytic) with subjects' self-ratings. Against the criterion of peer ratings on such variables as dominance, sociability, responsibility, and other similar characteristics, Hase and Goldberg reported that "in almost every case, the subjects' self-ratings were more predictive . . . than *any* of the scales (p. 245)." Even when linear regression equations were used to capitalize on the optimal combination of scales, self-prediction proved to be more accurate.

Relatively few studies have been carried out to compare the predictive ability of behavioral approaches to assessment with more traditional procedures. The limited data that are available, however, would seem to favor behavioral assessment.

CONCLUDING COMMENT

One of the basic characteristics of behavioral assessment is the attempt to maximize the similarity between test response and criterion measure. The desirability of approaching the prediction process in such a way so as to reduce the number of inferences has been argued by Cronbach (1956), who has observed:

> Assessment encounters trouble because it involves hazardous inferences. Very little inference is involved when a test is a sample of the criterion or when an empirical key is developed. Simple test interpretations involve inference from test to construct to behavioral prediction. But assessors attempt a maximum inference from tests. As current writers describe the process . . . . personality theory is applied to weave nomothetic constructs into a construct of the individual's personality structure; predictions are than derived by inferring how that structure will interact with the known or guessed properties of the situation. Assessors have been foolhardy to venture predictions of behavior in unanalyzed situations, using tests whose construct interpretations are dubious and personality theory which has more gaps than solid matter. (pp. 173-174)

While the successfully validated test provides support for the numerous assumptions involved in predicting criterion behaviors from test behavior, the unsuccessful effort at validation provides no clue to the weak link in the inference process. The analysis presented in this chapter suggests that any breakdown of the predictive powers of a test may productively be viewed as due to one or more inferences based on faulty assumptions concerning the measurement process and the phenomena of interest.

In the case of traditional personality tests, some of the basic underlying assumptions—such as the existence of behavioral consistencies across a wide variety of stimulus situations—have been found to be unsupported by empirical evidence. Other assumptions, such as those involving theoretical relationships hypothesized between test responses and constructs, are often vaguely stated or poorly defined, and consequently are difficult to test directly. The assessment of personality by means of behavioral tests, by contrast, is more consistent with the findings that human functioning is due to both the individual's behavioral repertoire and the demands of the specific stimulus situation. Further, relatively fewer assumptions are associated with this approach to test construction, and those that are involved can more readily be subjected to direct experimental investigation. By allowing for a more systematic elimination of erroneous inferences when validity coefficients are unsatisfactory, the behavioral approach to personality assessment would appear to have greater potential for the development of procedures that may enhance our ability to predict human behavior.

SUMMARY

In this chapter, the traditional and behavioral approaches to the prediction of human behavior have been examined with respect to such underlying assumptions as the basic conception of personality functioning, the selection of test items, and the interpretation of the responses to the test. Whereas traditional tests of personality involve the assessment of hypothesized personality constructs that, in turn, are used to predict overt behavior, the behavioral approach entails more of a direct sampling of the criterion behaviors themselves. In addition to requiring fewer inferences than traditional tests, behavioral assessment procedures have been described as being based on assumptions more amenable to direct empirical test and more consistent with empirical evidence. The available research findings on the comparative predictive ability of the two approaches similarly suggest that the behavioral orientation is a potentially useful approach toward the construction of assessment procedures that can more accurately predict human behavior.

4

Assessment of Semantic Schemas

The assessment of cognitive activities has a long and rich history, and is reflected in the pioneering efforts of such people as Binet, Cattell, Esquirol, Galton, Jung, Murray, Rorschach, and Sequin. The focus of this chapter, however, will deal with a much more recent stage in the history of cognitive assessment, namely the efforts that have been made by cognitive-behavior therapists through the early 1980s. Although some of the assessment procedures used by behavior therapists bear some similarity to those methods that have been used in the past, the point of divergence between behavioral and non-behavioral approaches can be found in the assumptions underlying both the construction and interpretation of behavioral assessment methods (see Chapters 2 and 3). Recognizing that behavior is a function of the situation as well as any enduring characteristics of the individual, behavioral assessors have been reluctant to measure global, trait-like tendencies. In marked contrast to the methodology inherent in projective techniques, where the nature of the situation is deliberately made to be ambiguous, behavioral assessors have taken care to clearly specify the nature of the situation as part of the assessment procedure. Because the essential unit of investigation consists not of an underlying personality construct but rather the individual's response to particular situations, the situational aspect of any assessment procedure becomes all important.

As behavior therapists began to recognize the relevance of cognition in the late 1960s and early 1970s, their interest was drawn to the task of cognitive assessment. It should be noted that this attention to cognitive variables did not come from an extrapolation from basic theory and research, but instead grew out of the clinical context. Although operant procedures were effective in dealing with chronic schizophrenics and young children, these methods were not found to be adequate in dealing with other populations. Consequently, the work of such individuals as Beck, Ellis, Lazarus, Mahoney, and Meichenbaum provides an important complement to existing behavioral interventions.

METHODS OF SAMPLING COGNITIONS

In 1958, George Kelly reviewed the available assessment techniques, which primarily consisted of indirect methods stemming from a psychodynamic orientation. As part of his review, Kelly made what at the time was a radical, but simple suggestion: "If you don't know what is going on in a person's mind, ask him; he may tell you" (p. 330). This, in essence, has been the overriding philosophy of the behavioral approach to the assessment of cognitions. Procedures for sampling cognitions have been administered *prior* to a task performance or social interaction (e.g., interviews, attribution questionnaires, measures of unrealistic beliefs, expectancy ratings); *during* the performance itself (e.g., think-aloud methods); or *following* the performance (e.g., thought listing, interviews, questionnaires) (Meichenbaum & Butler, 1980). As is the case with behavioral procedures in general, the sampling procedure is typically carried out within the context of a particular type or class of situations. For example, in a study by Cacioppo, Glass, and Merluzzi (1979), heterosocially anxious and nonanxious men were asked to list the thoughts they had immediately prior to engaging in an interaction with a woman. These thoughts were later rated by independent judges, revealing that in comparison to the nonanxious men, anxious subjects listed more negative and fewer positive self-statements before entering the social situation.

A wide variety of different assessment procedures have been developed over the years, measuring a number of different cognitive variables (e.g., expectancies, attributions, unrealistic beliefs). We will not deal with these in any comprehensive way, as detailed reviews of what is available may be found in existing books on the subject (e.g., Kendall & Hollon, 1981; Merluzzi, Glass & Genest, 1981). Instead, the purpose of this chapter is to draw on clinical experience as well as theory and research in experimental cognitive psychology to discuss those cognitive variables that may not be readily reported by clients or subjects, but which nonetheless serve as determinants of their thoughts, emotions, and behavior.

THE QUESTION OF AWARENESS

For those of us involved in cognitive assessment within the clinical context, the assessment of "internal dialogues" or what clients are "telling themselves" within any particular situation is not always as straightforward as it might seem. As noted in Chapter 1, what we are frequently interested in determining is not so much what clients are deliberately thinking, but rather the more elusive *meaning* that they may be assigning to any given event. Thus, even though clients may not be able to directly report certain cognitions, they may readily acknowledge that they are reacting emotionally or behaviorally "as if" they are saying certain things to themselves.

Within the experimental literature (e.g. Bower, 1975), it is generally acknowledged that human memory and meaning is associative in nature. In my own clinical attempts to assist clients in uncovering unrealistic thought patterns that may be mediating emotional distress, I have found the use of an associative task to be most helpful. Thus, instead of asking clients what they may be saying to themselves, associations to semi-structured incomplete sentences, such as "Making a mistake in front of my friends would upset me because . . ." can be most helpful. The similarity to Jung's early research (Jung, 1910) on the use of word associations to determine the idiosyncratically perceived significance of certain words is particularly striking. Keeping with a basic assumption underlying behavioral approaches to assessment, however, these associations are elicited within a specific situational context.

Most of the initial research and clinical work that has been done in cognitive-behavioral assessment has tended to deal with cognitive *products*—samples of the individual's thoughts in particular situations. It is only in more recent years that attempts have been made to assess the cognitive *processes* and *structures* that are reflected by these products (cf. Kihlstrom & Nasby, 1981; Landau & Goldfried, 1981). In doing so, cognitive behavior therapy has begun to draw on the work of experimental cognitive psychology.

EXTRAPOLATIONS FROM COGNITIVE PSYCHOLOGY

Research done by experimental cognitive psychologists has revealed that context plays a critical role in the meaning that individuals assign to events. For example, a study by Bransford and Johnson (1973) has shown how slight shifts in context can create dramatic changes in the meaning of an event. Consider the following passage:

> The man stood before the mirror and combed his hair. He checked his face carefully for any places he might have missed shaving and then put on the conservative tie he had decided to wear. At breakfast, he studied the newspaper carefully and, over coffee, discussed the possibility of buying a new washing machine with his wife. Then he made several phone calls. As he was leaving the house he thought about the fact that his children would probably want to go to that private camp again this summer. When the car didn't start, he got out, slammed the door and walked down to the bus stop in a very angry mood. Now he would be late. (p. 415)

If this passage would have begun with "the *unemployed* man stood before the mirror . . ." the meaning of the communication might be very different. As found by Branford and Johnson, change occurred not only in understanding of what events took place but also in the subject's inferences about why they did. Still a different meaning would emerge if the passage would begin with "the *stockbroker* stood before the mirror. . . ." If you were to read the passage once again, it would be evident that it takes on a different meaning if the person involved is unemployed or is a stockbroker.

The possibility of creating meaning shifts by virtue of changes in context can have important clinical implications. Take, for example, the case of a couple being seen in sex therapy. In this particular case, the wife had been the more sexually interested and active partner, with the husband tending to avoid sexual encounters for weeks and months at a time. After reviewing their sexual history as a couple, the therapist concluded that many of their past attempts to improve their sexual relations seemed to have been carried out within an adversarial context, in which the wife's job was to entice her reluctant husband into a sexual encounter; his role had been to resist. It was suggested that their between-session sexual activities be viewed within a more collaborative framework, in which they *both* were to work together to improve their sex lives. The husband was encouraged to increase the frequency of his sexual advances, not out of "pressure" but out of a desire to have a more satisfactory relationship with his wife. In the following week, he took the unprecedented step of initiating a sexual encounter not once but twice during the same week. During the second encounter, the wife decided to put on the flimsy negligee that her husband had bought her several years earlier, but which she had never before worn. In discussing their experiences during the next therapy session, the husband commented on the negligee, indicating that he was surprised that she decided to wear it after all these years. The wife then confessed that she had always resented the prospect of wearing it, as she viewed it as a reminder that her husband did not find her sexually attractive for herself. Because of what had gone on in the previous therapy session as well as her husband's second initiation during the course of the same week, she saw this recent sexual interaction as taking place within a more collaborate as opposed to adversarial context. Hence, wearing the negligee took on a radically different meaning for her — it was something that she could do to please him.

In talking about the use of a different context to create a meaning shift, we are in essence referring to a categorization process. Depending on the category in which a particular event gets placed, the meaning of the event is likely to differ. Indeed, the clinical effects of a procedure such as *reframing* may be understood in this light.

An increasing number of behavior therapists have proposed that an information processing model may be a particularly useful paradigm for understanding clinically relevant cognitive variables. This model, which has been particularly popular in experimental cognitive psychology for a number of years, postulates several nonconscious cognitive processes that operate both on incoming and stored information. Thus, when individuals interact with their environment, potential distortions may occur by virtue of selective attention, inappropriate classification of events, idiosyncratic storage of information, and/or inaccurate retrieval from memory.

The concept of *schema* has been suggested as being particularly useful in understanding this distortion process. In the most general sense, a schema refers to a cognitive representation of one's past experiences with situations or people, which eventually serves to assist individuals in constructing their perception of events within that domain. Although there are varying definitions of a schema, most reflect three basic assumptions

(Thorndyke & Hayes-Roth, 1979): First, a schema is said to involve an *organization* of conceptually related elements, representing a prototypical abstraction of a complex concept. From a clinical vantage point, these complex concepts are likely to consist of types of situations or types of persons. Specific examples are said to be stored in a schema, as well as the relationship among these examples. Second. a schema is *induced* from the "bottom-up," based on repeated past experiences involving many examples of the complex concept it represents. And finally, a schema is seen as *guiding* the organization of new information, much like a template or computer format allows for the attention to or processing of some information, but not others.

Among the advantages of the schema is that it can facilitate learning and the recognition, recall, and comprehension of information that is schema-relevant. It allows us to chunk information into larger, more meaningful units—so-called "knowledge structures"—giving a sense of meaning to the world around us. It also helps us to fill in the gaps when there is missing information, and provides us with greater confidence in making predictions about the world around us. At the same time, these advantages can serve as liabilities, particularly if a schema is no longer relevant to one's current life situation. In essence, our past interactions with the world have provided us with propensities to view the world — or ourselves — in given ways, even though these perceptions may no longer be valid.

Many of the cognitive variables that we sample directly with our assessment procedures may be construed as a product of semantic schemas, or the characteristic ways individuals attribute meaning to those situations, individuals, objects, and actions that impact on their lives. What individuals tell themselves in particular situations only accompany, and are a result of, the person's perception of the situations, which depends in part on the semantic schemas that he or she may bring to bear in encoding the situation.

THE MEASUREMENT OF SEMANTIC SCHEMAS

Of all the techniques for the assessment of semantic schemas, word associations have been used the longest (Deese, 1965). Within the experimental literature, word association procedures have been viewed as providing a potentially useful index of meaning (Nobel, 1952). As cognitive psychology has developed over the years, varying types of association methods have been employed. In the clinical setting, however, associative methods have typically been the province of psychodynamic approaches. Nonetheless, if we define a behavioral approach to clinical work as involving the extrapolation from the experimental literature, it is important that we examine the relevance of the associative procedures used in experimental psychology—even if our past tendency may have been to classify association methods as belonging to a psychodynamic orientation.

One method that has been used to evaluate semantic schemas consists of *attribute-listing*, an associative procedure whereby individuals enumerate as many attributes or features as possible in a given amount of time (Fishbein & Ajzen, 1975). These procedures are based on the assumption that objects are represented in semantic memory by a prototype, consisting of a list of those attributes that belong to the particular class of objects. In recognizing or classifying any object or situation, its attributes are matched against these internal prototypes to find the prototype that best characterizes the stimulus in question.

Attribute-listing procedures have been used in a variety of different ways. For example, Cantor, Mischel, and Schwartz (1982) have used this procedure for developing a taxonomy of interpersonal situations as perceived by the ordinary person. The clinical relevance of this methodology is particularly intriguing, as distortions or misconceptions of upsetting objects, people, actions, or situations can be understood in terms of an attribute-sampling model, The particular way an event or object is categorized depends on those attributes that are encoded, which is presumably a function or tendency of schemas to direct a person's attention to particular attributes. For example, dog phobics, when compared with nonphobics, have been found to list attributes associated with dogs that tend to be less pleasant (Landau, 1980). Similarly, when socially anxious males are asked to give attributes that they associate with a typical interaction with a female, they list significantly more unpleasant attributes than do nonanxious individuals. (Goldfried, Padawer & Robins, 1984).

Another method that may be used for the assessment of schematic schemas is the Semantic Differential (Osgood, Suci, & Tannenbaum, 1957). This procedure involves having individuals rate a number of preselected concepts on several seven-point bipolar rating scales, such as strong-weak, good-bad, fast-slow, etc. Numerous studies with a variety of different concepts, and across different settings, have typically yielded the dimensions of evaluation, potency, and activity. This procedure can lend itself particularly well to a number of clinical questions, as it is possible to determine the extent to which different concepts that are rated—be they individuals or situations—are perceived by clients as being semantically similar from their particular vantage point.

Still another procedure that has been used quite frequently for investigating semantic schemas is multidimensional scaling (Carroll & Arabie, 1980). Unlike the semantic differential, which consists of ratings obtained across dimensions of evaluation, potency and activity, multidimensional scaling allows for the possible uncovering of the unique implicit dimensions that individuals use when they classify or make perceived similarity judgments about various people, events, objects, or situations. Multidimensional scaling makes use of an individual's judgment of similarity between different concepts, which can be obtained in a number of different ways. It may entail ratings of similarity among all concepts (e.g. similarity ratings between "boss" and "father," "boss" and "friend," "father" and "friend"), or may simply involve the sorting of concepts into what people believe to be meaningful categories. The procedure is somewhat similar to factor analytic methods, and the degree of similarity between varying concepts can be represented visually by their distance from each other in n-dimensional space.

There is a form of multidimensional scaling—INDSCAL (Carroll & Chang, 1970)—that has been found to be particularly useful in studying clinically-related phenomena. Not only does it allow one to uncover underlying implicit dimensions that are used in the classification process—the "categories-in-the-head"—but it can also detect individual differences in the tendencies to make use of these dimensions. In a study comparing dog phobics and non-phobics, Landau (1980) used INDSCAL in analyzing similarity ratings of various types of dogs and other mammals. The two primary dimensions revealed in the similarity ratings consisted of size and dangerousness. In the case of judgments of mammals, the phobics and non-phobics did not differ in their use of these two dimensions. In judging the similarity among dogs, however, phobics tended to overemphasize the dangerousness dimension, whereas non-phobics used both size and dangerousness more comparably. Thus, the dog schema for phobic individuals reflected their greater tendency to classify these animals particularly in terms of their potential danger.

We have extended this methodology in our study of socially anxious college men (Goldfried et al., 1984), so as to determine how they differ from non-anxious men in the classification of social situations. Subjects were divided into two extreme groups on the basis of their heterosocial anxiety scores on the Situation Questionnaire (Rehm & Marston, 1968), a paper-and-pencil measure designed to determine anxiety levels in varying types of heterosocial interactions. They were then given thirty index cards, each containing a description of a heterosocial situation contained within the questionnaire itself, and were asked to visualize each as clearly as possible and then to arrange them in categories on the basis of similarity. They had the option to use as many categories as they wished and also to include as many or as few situations as they would like in any given category. After having done this sorting, they again were given the opportunity to look over the cards in each pile one more time to make any final adjustments. The average number of categories used by both the high-and low-anxious subjects did not differ significantly. To determine the degree of similarity among all possible pairs of situations and thereby to understand the underlying cognitive dimensions on which the similarity judgments were based, the sorting data were compiled into matrices for both groups by determining the number of subjects in each group that sorted any given pair of situations together. The particular multidimensional scaling procedure used (INDSCAL) not only indicated the degree of similarity perceived among the various situations, but also revealed the relative emphasis given by the high and low socially anxious groups to each of the obtained dimensions.

The results revealed three separate dimensions, each of which was interpreted on the basis of the situations located at different points on each dimension. Thus, in the case of the first dimension—*intimacy*—at one end there were such items as "kissing a girl good-night at the door," "dancing with a girl on a date," and other situations related to dating. At the other end of the first dimension were such situations as "talking to a girl with a group of male and female friends" and "casually talking to a girl much younger than yourself." The second dimension—*chance of being evaluated*—reflected social interactions that held the potential for being evaluated by the woman. Thus, at one end there were such items as "being introduced to a new girl at a party" and "starting a conversation with a girl whom you have never met before in dorm lounge or cafeteria," and at the other extreme were such situations as "calling a girl for information about a class" and "talking to an older woman whom you know." The third dimension — *academic relevance* — appeared to reflect whether the interaction was related to school issues, such as "asking a girl for information about a class" versus "casually talking to a girl much younger than yourself".

The weighting for each of these three dimensions was obtained separately for high and low socially anxious individuals. What the dimension weight essentially tells us is the extent to which the particular group relies on a given dimension in evaluating the perceived similarity of these social situations. For men who *did not* experience anxiety in these social situations, the degree of intimacy associated with these various interactions was the most dominant category used. That is, they tended to make distinctions among these situations primarily on the basis of whether or not they were associated with intimacy. Of the three dimensions, these non-anxious men were *least likely* to make use of "the chance of being evaluated" as an implicit category. Anxious men, on the other hand, used chance of being evaluated to the same degree as intimacy in categorizing these social situations. Finally, the "academic relevance" category was used least by the socially anxious subjects, which may be interpreted as reflecting the difficulty anxious individuals have in focusing on the external cues of a social interaction and its associated response requirements.

Other procedures for assessing semantic schemas, such as those devised by Rosenberg (1977), may be used for an individual case. To do this the person first prepares a list of a number of individuals in their lives and a list of traits and feelings associated with each of them. Each of the individuals are then rated on the basis of the trait and feeling characteristics, which can then be subjected to a hierarchical cluster analysis. The results of all of this is a hierarchically organized depiction of the similarities and differences among these individuals as perceived by the particular subject.

Any discussion of the assessment of semantic structure would be incomplete without note of Kelly's (1955) Rep test and related grid techniques, which have proven to be most useful clinically in the characterization of interpersonal relationships. In actuality it is not a single test, but rather a more general type of methodology whereby a number of "elements" (e.g. names of significant others in one's life) are grouped according to similarities and differences along certain dimensions. The various applications of this procedure have been extensively reviewed by Neimeyer and Neimeyer (1981) and Thomas and Harri-Augstein (1985).

SUMMARY

As behavior therapists began to recognize the relevance of cognition, their interest was drawn to the task of cognitive assessment. A wide variety of procedures have been developed for sampling cognitions. either prior to entering a situation during performance itself or afterwards. Most of the initial research and clinical work that has been done in cognitive-behavioral assessment has tended to deal with cognitive products—samples of the individual's thoughts in particular situations. It is only in more recent years that attempts have been made to assess the cognitive processes and structures that are reflected by these products. In doing so, cognitive behavior therapy has begun to draw on the work of experimental cognitive psychology.

The chapter has discussed the role of context in contributing to the meaning individuals attribute to events, and examples were given from the experimental literature as well as clinical experience. The concept of schema was suggested as a way of understanding the potential distortions that may occur when an individual interacts with the environment, by virtue of selective attention, inappropriate classification of events, idiosyncratic storage of information, and/or inaccurate retrieval from memory. The chapter also described a variety of different means by which semantic schemas may be assessed.

The possibility of uncovering and altering an individual's hierarchically arranged semantic structures for various classes of life events is an intriguing, if not challenging prospective. Behavior therapy has a tradition of therapeutic intervention that emphasizes "bottom-up" change, in the sense of altering an individual's reactions to specific situations. By contrast, the psychodynamic tradition has tended to focus on "top-down" change, assuming that behavior change will follow the growing awareness of one's faulty cognitive structures. As cognitive-behavior therapy becomes increasingly more influenced by experimental cognitive psychology and social cognition, intervention procedures are likely to be developed that make use of *both* "top-down" and "bottom-up" change (Goldfried & Robins, 1983).

Part III
A COGNITIVE-BEHAVIORAL APPROACH TO FACILITATING COPING SKILLS

Perhaps more than any other therapeutic orientation, cognitive-behavior therapy has directly confronted the issue of control as it exists within the therapy relationship. Cognitive-behavior therapists begin by assuming that clients enter treatment because of their inability to deal with the difficulties that they have in life, and are requesting assistance and direction in order to help ameliorate these problems. Consequently, the behavioral orientation provides a clinical atmosphere that endorses therapeutic guidance and directiveness. Because of this philosophical stance, behavior therapy was frequently criticized in the 1960s and early 1970s for "manipulating" clients' behavior and paying only minimal attention to assisting them in developing methods for independently dealing with their own lives.

In reality, behavior therapists, like therapists of other theoretical orientations, have always been mindful of the need to help clients deal with their own lives. Even in the classic debate between Rogers and Skinner (1956), both agreed that there are dangers associated with the control of human behavior. They also both acknowledged the desirability of assisting clients in obtaining a sense of self-direction. The essential difference between Rogers and Skinner had to do with the *means* by which this goal might be accomplished, with behavior therapists having a greater willingness to be more directive in their interventions.

In an early formulation dealing with methods for providing clients with a sense of self-control, Bandura (1969) referred to this process as involving a form of reciprocal interaction. Thus, while acknowledging that reinforcement contingencies can significantly influence an individual's behavior, Bandura suggested that cognitive processes may greatly enhance the change process by assisting clients in becoming more aware of the contingencies that govern their own behavior. To the extent that clients are able to use their cognitive capacities to evaluate the determinants of their functioning, they are in a better position to make the types of changes in their lives that might lead to a more optimal state of functioning. This formulation led Goldfried and Merbaum (1973) to offer a definition of self control as involving *"a personal decision arrived at through conscious deliberation for the purpose of integrating action which is designed to achieve certain desired outcomes or goals as determined by the individual himself"* (p. 12).

The early work done in behavior therapy under the rubric of "self-control" gave way in the 1980s to a view of therapy as providing a vehicle for training clients in "coping skills." In many respects, the term "coping skills" is better suited to describing what is involved in the therapeutic procedures themselves, in that it does not imply a constraint of impulses, and more clearly connotes that a learning process is involved. Precisely *what* is learned goes beyond a specific solution to a particular problem, and instead involves cognitive and behavioral methods that individuals can use for dealing with types of difficult situations in their lives. The coping skills notion of intervention also implies that the therapist is less of a healer and more of a teacher, consultant, and supervisor who works with clients in a collaborate fashion in helping to teach them how to function more effectively—in essence, to act as their own therapists.

The first selection in this section provides a conceptualization of systematic desensitization as a method for helping clients learn to cope with anxiety. The coping skill is essentially that of relaxation, which is used not so much as a passive method for reconditioning, but rather a procedure that individuals may use to reduce their anxiety in a wide variety of different situations. Interestingly enough, the original description of relaxation training by Jacobson (1929) presented it in very much this way. For a variety of different practical and theoretical reasons — there were no tape recorders available for at-home practice, and it did easily fit into the prevailing psychoanalytic model of change — relaxation initially made relatively little impact on the field. As a result of Wolpe's ingenious utilization of relaxation for purposes of systematic desensitization some 30 years later (Wolpe, 1958), its clinical utility began to become more widely recognized.

The use of relaxation within a context of systematic desensitization was for purposes of passively deconditioning individuals to different fearful situations. Indeed, early research to determine the effectiveness of desensitization concluded that relaxation training by itself was not clinically effective. It was only as a result of ongoing clinical work in this area that it became more apparent relaxation training could often be used in and of itself for purposes of anxiety reduction. In Chapter 5, both conceptual and procedural modifications of systematic desensitization are described, such that it can be more appropriately construed as a rehearsal procedure that helps to teach clients in using relaxation as an active coping skill.

However useful relaxation may be for helping individuals to cope with anxiety, there are often instances where its effectiveness may be undermined. This would occur particularly in those circumstances where an individual's emotional arousal (i.e. anxiety, depression, anger) is cognitively mediated. Thus, while an individual may be momentarily successful in reducing anxiety by means of relaxation, he or she may unwittingly undermine these beneficial effects by cognitive mediation (e.g. "I really *have* to perform extremely well in this situation, otherwise something terrible will happen").

Chapter 6 describes a method for helping individuals reduce their anxiety by learning to reevaluate more realistically the potentially threatening events in their lives. These therapeutic guidelines were based on the work of Ellis (1962), who has argued — often vigorously — that the way individuals perceive situations plays an important role in creating their problems. In essence, Ellis has suggested that faulty labeling has its basis in certain unrealistic beliefs, such as the excessive need for approval from others and the belief that one needs to perform all things perfectly. Ellis's rational-emotive therapy is designed to help individuals think more logically and reevaluate these and other erroneous beliefs. In providing these guidelines for rational restructuring, my goal was to depart from Ellis's contention that the most effective way to help clients learn to think more realistically was by vigorous and repeated presentations of realistic thinking. Instead, I suggested that a more systematic approach may be used to help individuals in this learning process. In many way, it parallels the suggestions made in Chapter 5 on the use of systematic desensitization as a coping skill, except that instead of coping by means of the relaxation response, realistic reappraisal is used as the active coping skill.

In Chapter 7, taken from an article written together with Clive Robins, we provide a conceptualization of and guidelines for helping clients update their sense of self-worth. This selection was written in response to the traditional behavioral assumption that individuals tend to be fairly logical in processing their therapeutic gains, and that all the therapist needed to do was to help them behave differently. With more experience in the clinical practice of behavior therapy, it became apparent to an increasing number of clinicians that the change process was not nearly so straightforward, and clients often showed signs of resistance. Even when they showed overt behavioral changes, they nonetheless tended to be slow in changing the views they had about themselves. This typically takes the form of "Yes-butting" therapeutic progress away, where the therapeutic gains may be forgotten or in some other way discounted.

Although this tendency on the part of clients to deny their therapeutic progress may be a great source of frustration to therapists, a review of the experimental cognitive psychology literature suggests that it is to be expected. Schemas—either about others or oneself—are notoriously difficult to change, even when one's life circumstance indicates that change has indeed occurred. The purpose of the last chapter in this section is to consider why clients have such difficulties in recognizing changes in their lives, particularly the problems they have in updating their views of themselves. It deals with the general concept of self-mastery, and describes how the field of cognitive psychology can help us better understand the self-deceptive processes that can undermine therapeutic progress. It also provides therapeutic guidelines on how to help clients bring about changes in their self-schemas.

5

Systematic Desensitization as Training in Self-Control

The specific procedures traditionally employed in systematic desensitization follow logically from the theoretical description of the treatment process as outlined by Wolpe (1958). According to the principle of reciprocal inhibition, Wolpe maintains:

> If a response antagonistic to anxiety can be made to occur in the presence of anxiety-evoking stimuli so that it is accompanied by a complete or partial suppression of the anxiety responses, the bond between these stimuli and the anxiety responses will be weakened. (p. 71)

Although research evidence clearly indicates that systematic desensitization does indeed work, one can nonetheless call into question the adequacy of Wolpe's theoretical explanation for the underlying process. For example, it has yet to be demonstrated that relaxation functions in the way in which Wolpe suggests, namely, as a response that is inherently antagonistic to anxiety (Lang, 1969). An even more basic assumption underlying Wolpe's theory—and one toward which the present chapter addresses itself—is that the relearning that occurs during the treatment sessions represents a relatively passive process of deconditioning. As indicated below, it would seem more appropriate to construe systematic desensitization as more of an active process, directed toward learning of a general anxiety-reducing skill, rather than the passive desensitization to specific aversive stimuli.

Following the description of a mediational model to explain the effectiveness of desensitization, and a discussion of some of the corroborative research findings for this alternative explanation, specific

67

procedural modifications for systematic desensitization will be suggested.

A MEDIATIONAL INTERPRETATION

Rather than viewing relaxation as "reciprocally inhibiting" the anxiety reaction, a mediational conceptualization of desensitization would instead describe the situation as follows: Because of the individual's previous life experiences, he or she has learned to react to certain environmental situations with an avoidance response. Further, this overt response may be conceptualized as being the end product of a series of mediational responses and stimuli. According to this view, one can maintain that systematic desensitization involves not so much a passive "reciprocal inhibition" as it does the *active building in of the muscular relaxation response and cognitive relabeling into the mediational sequence.*

During the process of systematic desensitization, clients are taught to become sensitive to their proprioceptive cues for tension, and to react to these cues with their newly acquired skill in muscular relaxation. They are also taught to differentiate the proprioceptive feedback associated with tension from that associated with relaxation, and to identify this feeling of "calm" with the state of muscular relaxation. Once clients have been successful in reducing muscular tension and experiencing the feeling of calm in the aversive situation, they are in a better position to approach, rather than avoid, the heretofore fearful object. According to this view, then, what clients learn is a means of actively coping with the anxiety, rather than an immediate replacement for it.

With further practice — both in the consultation session and in vivo — clients become better able to identify their proprioceptive cues for muscular tension, to respond by voluntarily relaxing it away, and to relabel their emotional state accordingly (cf. Schachter & Singer, 1962). As this learning proceeds still further, relaxation responses may become anticipatory, thereby completely or partially "short circuiting" the anxiety reaction. In line with Osgood's (1953) discussion of mediation, one might also expect that with repeated practice of the mediational sequence, the responses and cues that initially have been proprioceptive would continue, but at a cortical level.

Supporting Evidence

There are a number of findings that can more readily be explained by a mediational model than by the counterconditioning hypothesis (Goldfried, 1979). For example, in an attempt to look for possible symptom substitution accompanying successful desensitization, several studies (Lang & Lazovik, 1963; Lang et al., 1965; Paul, 1966; Paul & Shannon, 1966) report that in marked contrast to the possible emergence of new fears, individuals tend to report a general decrement in fearfulness. Of particular importance is the fact that this generalized anxiety reduction occurs with respect to objects or situations that differ widely as to their stimulus properties—a finding that is not easily explained by the stimulus generalization that is likely to follow from the counter-conditioning of specific fears. On the other hand, these findings are quite consistent with the hypothesis that successful desensitization results in the learning of a more generalized anxiety-reducing skill, which individuals learn to apply at times they experience tension.

Some studies have noted that although anxiety reduction does indeed occur during the desensitization sessions themselves, the amount of transfer to real-life situations is not complete (Agras, 1967; Davison, 1968; Lang & Lazovik, 1963; Lang et al., 1965). Thus, although they are better able to approach the previously feared objects, successfully desensitized individuals nonetheless do report experiencing tension. Although it may be possible to explain this lack of perfect transfer by referring to the discrepancies between the situations presented in imagination and those occurring in real life (Davison, 1968), Agras' (1967) interpretation of these findings seems more plausible. Agras suggests that there may be two phases that account for the successful results achieved with systematic desensitization: the learning that occurs during the desensitization sessions themselves and the changes that occur *in vivo*. This view of desensitization is very much in accord with the mediational paradigm described above, where the treatment procedure provides the client with a technique for coping with anxiety that may be expected to prevent (i.e., short circuit) anxiety only after it is fully learned by repeated trials in the real-life situation.

In an attempt to determine the necessary and sufficient procedural conditions for anxiety reduction through systematic desensitization, researchers have consistently found that relaxation training per se appears to have little effect on subjects (Davison, 1968; Lang et al., 1965; Rachman, 1965). At first blush, these findings appear to contradict the mediational interpretation of desensitization. Inasmuch as the people in these investigations were simply trained in relaxation and never really instructed in how or when to use this response, however, the role of relaxation in systematic desensitization was studied only in a limited sense. In addition to clinical reports (e.g., Davison, 1965; D'Zurilla, 1969; Gray, England, & Mohoney, 1965) attesting to the effectiveness of relaxation used *in vivo*, Zeisset (1968) has presented some empirical findings consistent with these clinical observations. After training subjects in relaxation, Zeisset instructed them to "use" this newly acquired skill in everyday life whenever they began to experience tension. In contrast to previous studies indicating that relaxation alone was not effective in reducing anxiety, it was found that relaxation training plus the instruction to apply this technique when anxious was more successful in reducing anxiety in the criterion situation (i.e., "interview anxiety") than placebo and no-contact controls, and just as effective as systematic desensitization that used criterion-relevant hierarchy.

The work on the use of drug-induced (methohexitone sodium or Brevital) relaxation in systematic desensitization provides some findings that appear to be consistent with a mediational, self-control model. Commenting on the variable results others have had in utilizing Brevital to induce states of relaxation, Brady (1967) has suggested that an important procedural detail for the successful use of the drug involves instructions that clients "work along with it" and allow themselves to relax. Davison and Valins (1968) have similarly noted the importance of having clients "let go" even when drugs are being used to aid in the induction of muscular relaxation, so that the success in relaxation can be attributed, at least in part, to their own efforts. From this point of view, effective fear reduction follows from an active attempt on the part of clients to relax themselves rather than simply presenting aversive stimuli when individuals happen to be in a state of relaxation.

In discussing the possible role of cognitive variables in desensitization, Lang (1969) has hypothesized that clients may be learning a "cognitive set" regarding their emotional arousal, whereby

desensitization is an operant training schedule, designed to shape the response "I am not afraid" (or a potentially competing response such as

"I am relaxed" or "I am angry") in the presence of a graded set of discriminative stimuli. When well learned, the response could have the status of a "set" or self-instruction, which can then determine other related behaviors . . . . (p. 187)

Lang's suggestion that such learning may be inadvertently reinforced by the therapist (and client's themselves), as well as the finding by Leitenberg et al. (1969) that the systematic reinforcement of the individual's progress during systematic desensitization facilitates improvement, further supports the hypothesis that desensitization is actually providing the client with an active coping skill.

It is of considerable interest to note that even with the therapist viewing systematic desensitization as a counterconditioning of specific fears, clients often perceive the beneficial effects of treatment as their having learned a strategy for coping with stress in general. For example, in their study on the effects of group desensitization, Paul and Shannon (1966) report that

subjects in the group seemed to perceive the desensitization method as an active mastery technique which they could acquire and use themselves, more than in the individual application. Clients' descriptions of utilizing desensitization training to master anticipated areas of stress themselves suggest the development of a confidence-building "how to cope" orientation. (pp. 133–134)

The frequently noted generalized improvement resulting from systematic desensitization, which can be more readily explained with a self-control model, would certainly attest to the possibility that desensitization results in the learning of a generally applicable stress-reducing strategy.

Although a mediational, self-control view of systematic desensitization may be used to explain what goes on during the treatment process, the intent of this chapter is not simply to provide an alternative theoretical paradigm. The author agrees with Bandura (1961) that behavioral principles should not be used solely to explain currently available treatment methods, but rather to generate innovative, more effective procedures. It is toward a description of certain suggested procedural modifications that the next section is directed.

SUGGESTED PROCEDURAL MODIFICATIONS

Based on a mediational model of desensitization, as well as the supporting evidence for this general self-control orientation, several modifications in technique would appear to be indicated. These suggested procedural changes, the effectiveness of which are amenable to empirical test, include (a) a different rationale for systematic desensitization given to the client; (b) a different focus placed on the purpose of relaxation training; (c) different guidelines used in the construction of the hierarchy; (d) a modified manner in which the scenes are presented in imagination; and (e) a greater emphasis on instruction in the use of relaxation responses *in vivo*.

Rationale Presented to the Client

In structuring the therapeutic procedures for the client by describing the underlying rationale for desensitization, the following can be explained:

> There are various situations where, on the basis of your past experience, you have learned to react by becoming tense (anxious, nervous, fearful). What I plan to do is help you to learn how to cope with these situations more successfully, so that they do not make you as upset. This will be done by taking note of a number of those situations that upset you to varying degrees, and then having you learn to cope with the less stressful situations before moving on to the more difficult ones.
>
> Part of the treatment involves learning how to relax, so that in situations where you feel yourself getting nervous you will be better able to eliminate this tenseness. Learning to relax is much like learning any other skill. When you first learned to drive, you initially may have had difficulty in coordinating everything, and often found yourself very much aware of what you were doing. With more and more practice, however, the procedures involved in driving became easier and more automatic. You may find the same thing occurring to you when you try to relax in those situations where you feel yourself starting to become tense. You will find that as you persist, however, it will become easier and easier.

The general procedures of relaxation training, hierarchy construction, and successive presentation of items for imagination are then described to the client, with the additional indication that the purpose of the desensitization sessions is (a) to provide practice in learning to "relax away" tensions as they start to build up, and (b) to provide rehearsal for certain specific situations where the client may actually try out his relaxation skills *in vivo*.

Focus Placed on Relaxation Training

As a fairly representative method of relaxation training typically used in desensitization, we may note the procedure outlined by Paul (1966). This technique simply involves having the client tense separate muscle groups for approximately 5–7 seconds, taking note of the muscles that are tense, relaxing them for 20–30 seconds, and focusing on the sensations that are associated with relaxation.

The suggested modification of this procedure is slight and involves informing the clients that (a) the tension phase is provided so that they can be aware of those sensations that are involved in being tense, and (b) these sensations will serve as a signal or cue for them to relax away the tension—as they will be doing during the training sessions and *in vivo*. As they become better able to relax themselves using the tension relaxation procedure, they are given training in identifying the already-present tensions of which they may be aware, and then relaxing these away. Hence, in addition to learning a relaxation response, this phase of the desensitization procedure also provides the client with practice in recognizing the proprioceptive feedback associated with tension so it can serve as a cue for the appropriate use of relaxation.

Guideline for Hierarchy Construction

In the construction of the hierarchy, the typical approach used in desensitization involves a selection of graded variations of anxiety-provoking situations that reflect a given theme. Wolpe and Lazarus (1966) have also noted that there may be times when systematic desensitization would involve several themes, but that separate hierarchies should be compiled for each.

In using a mediational interpretation of desensitization, the nature of the specific environmental situation eliciting the anxiety becomes less important than the tension response itself. According to a mediational paradigm, *clients are being taught to cope with their proprioceptive anxiety responses and cues rather than with situations that elicit the tension.* What is being suggested here, then, is that the typical practice of establishing hierarchies that reflect carefully selected themes may not be essential to the successful application of systematic desensitization. Inasmuch as clients are being trained to relax away anxiety as it begins to build up, one need only construct a single hierarchy composed of situations eliciting increasing amounts of anxiety, irrespective of whether or not the items appear to reflect any given theme. In fact, the therapist might choose to select items that reflect a variety of different anxiety-producing situations in the individual's current life in order to facilitate generalization of the effect of desensitization. This would be particularly indicated in cases where the client responds with anxiety in a variety of different situations.

Presentation of Scenes in Imagination

During the course of the systematic desensitization itself, the therapist typically asks clients to visualize the scene for approximately 10–15 seconds, provided there is no anxiety response. Should clients indicate that they are beginning to feel tense, they are usually instructed to stop imagining the scene and concentrate only on trying to relax. This procedure is based on the assumption that in order to effect a successful counterconditioning, the relaxation response must be stronger than the anxiety response. Based on a mediational interpretation, however, clients would *not* be told to eliminate the scene once they begin to feel tense. In real life, clients cannot always remove themself from a situation once they start becoming anxious. By viewing the desensitization session as a rehearsal for anxiety reduction in specific real-life situations, as well as practice in successfully coping with anxiety in general, it would follow logically that clients should *maintain the image even though they are experiencing anxiety, and additionally to relax away this tension.* By using this approach, one more realistically parallels potentially stressful life situations, thereby providing clients with practice in modifying the mediational sequence. On the basis of the clinical experience of the author and several of his colleagues in the routine utilization of this procedure (e.g., D'Zurilla, 1969), this modification of desensitization has proven to be quite successful.

Use of Relaxation In Vivo

In accordance with the view of systematic desensitization as self-control training for the reduction of anxiety, clients should be encouraged to practice this skill *in vivo*. Thus, clients are told to identify their feelings of tension, to instruct themself to "relax" (cf. Bond & Hutchison, 1960; Cautela, 1966; D'Zurilla, 1969), and then actually to "let go" of their muscles. Although the utilization of relaxation *in vivo* may parallel some of the items in the desensitization hierarchy, it may also involve situations that were not incorporated into the hierarchy. Indeed, I have been struck with the success that some clients report in relaxing away tension in situations never discussed during therapy (e.g., one client who was being desensitized for speech anxiety found that the use of relaxation *in vivo* was instrumental in improving his golf game!). In encouraging clients to practice anxiety reduction *in vivo*, they should be forewarned that at times they may experience some difficulty in being completely successful at relaxing away tension. This would be particularly the case in those instances where the anxiety reaction is intense.

SUMMARY

The concept of self-control appears to be playing an increasingly significant role in the understanding and modification of a variety of different forms of maladaptive behavior. In accordance with a self-control orientation, this chapter has presented a mediational model of systematic desensitization, together with some of the procedural implications that follow from this formulation. Thus, rather than constructing desensitization as involving a more or less passive elimination of specific fears, the therapeutic procedure is seen as being directed toward providing clients with a more general skill for reducing anxiety, thereby enabling them to exercise greater self-control in a variety of anxiety-provoking life situations. Clinical experience and some empirical evidence would suggest that this alternative view with its procedural modifications is potentially quite fruitful.

6

Application of Rational Restructuring to Anxiety Disorders

> We shall not cease from exploration
> And the end of all our exploring
> Will be to arrive where we started
> And know the place for the first time.
>
> — T. S. Eliot

As noted earlier, the work done in behavior therapy in the late 1950s and 1960s ultimately led to the incorporation of cognitive variables in the conceptualization and remediation of a wide variety of clinical problems. Due in large part to the efforts of a number of therapists and researchers in what came to be known in the 1970s as "cognitive-behavior therapy" (Bandura, 1969; Beck, 1970; Goldfried, Decenteceo, & Weinberg, 1974; Kanfer & Phillips, 1970; Lazarus, 1971; Mahoney, 1974; Meichenbaum, 1974; Thoresen & Mahoney, 1974), it is now rare to find behavior therapists who do not acknowledge the relevance of cognitive variables in the therapeutic change process.

As noted by Meichenbaum (1977), however, one should be wary of the "uniformity myth" that suggests all cognitive-behavior therapy interventions are the same, including those that focus specifically on anxiety. The purpose of this chapter is not to review the different cognitive-behavioral procedures for anxiety reduction, but rather to describe in some detail one such procedure, namely rational restructuring. The general theoretical model and relevant research findings for this method will be outlined, followed by a detailed description of how the procedure may be implemented in clinical practice. I will also note the types of clients for which rational restructuring is particularly well suited.

THEORETICAL MODEL AND RESEARCH BASE

It has long been acknowledged that individuals' assumptions and expectations about the world around them can have profound implications for their emotional reaction and actual behavior. To the extent that people label a given situation "dangerous," their emotional and behavioral response to that situation will radically differ from other events that are labeled "safe." This, in itself, has relatively little clinical significance. Of greater importance is whether or not this labeling process is accurate or fallacious. To the extent that individuals are responding to a situation that they mislabel as dangerous — a point clearly articulated by Ellis (1962) — the treatment of choice would be to alter the labeling process more than the response to it.

Theoretical Model

With increased clinical experience in the use of cognitive-behavioral procedures, it became apparent to many workers in the field that clients were not always aware of how they construed various anxiety-related situations. Although many individuals may be able to report what they said to themselves in various anxiety-related situations (e.g., "I am concerned I may look foolish"), they were not always aware of the "underlying" reasons that this would be upsetting to them. The general belief by most workers in this area (e.g., Beck, Davison, Ellis, Goldfried, Lazarus, Mahoney, Meichenbaum) is that such "self-statements" are reflections of more basic assumptions, some of which may be tacit in nature.

As I have argued in earlier chapters, these tacit assumptions may be usefully construed as reflecting basic "schemas," which are the underlying assumptions that anxious individuals bring to a variety of different life events. Two such basic schemas one typically finds in routine clinical practice are those reflecting the need for *approval* from others (e.g., "If I am not liked and approved of by others, then I am no good"), and *perfection* (e.g., "If I don't do a perfect job in everything I attempt, then I'm a failure"). As will be seen in the presentation of the clinical procedures for the implementation of rational restructuring. considerable clinical skill is often needed in order to assist clients in identifying such schemas.

In a fascinating book entitled *Misunderstandings of the Self*, Raimy (1975) has suggested that most forms of therapy are directed toward assisting individuals in changing certain "misconceptions" that they may have about themselves or others. The task of the therapist, according to Raimy, is to assist clients in examining "evidence" that can help them to change their misconceptions. This may be accomplished in a variety of ways, such as discussion, explanations by the therapist, observing others, or through direct experience. Regardless of the procedure, however. clients must be able to step back and observe their misconceptions in light of this contradictory evidence. This therapeutic principle is central to rational restructuring.

Research Base

There have been a number of basic research findings that corroborate the theoretical assumptions described above, particularly the mediating role of cognitions. Because of space limitations, however, these findings will not be reviewed here; the interested reader can obtain reviews of these findings in a variety of sources (e.g., Goldfried, 1979; Meichenbaum, 1977; Merluzzi, Glass, & Genest, 1981; Smith, 1982). Most relevant to this chapter, however, is the research that has been carried out on the clinical effectiveness of rational restructuring.

In considering the research conducted on rational restructuring, it should be kept in mind that it is only one of several cognitive-behavioral procedures for anxiety reduction on which data have been obtained. A more comprehensive review of research in this area may be found elsewhere (e.g., Hollon & Beck, 1986; Kendell & Kriss, 1983). With regard to rational restructuring per se, outcome research has been conducted on such problems as social anxiety, unassertiveness, public speaking anxiety, test-taking anxiety, and Type A behavior. In addition, some work has been done on the application of this procedure to problems of anger, and a case report that demonstrated its application to bulimia.

In a study by Kanter and Goldfried (1979), socially anxious individuals were treated with rational restructuring, in which they learned to identify and reevaluate their anxiety-producing evaluations of social situations. When compared with self-control desensitization, rational restructuring demonstrated significant anxiety reduction. Other research findings have similarly demonstrated a tendency for rational restructuring to be more effective than desensitization in the treatment of social anxiety (Malkiewich & Merluzzi, 1980; Shahar & Merbaum, 1981).

Conceptualizing unassertive behavior as involving a component of social-evaluative anxiety, Linehan, Goldfried, and Goldfried (1979) determined that rational restructuring alone was able to reduce the inhibiting effects of anxiety and consequently increase assertive behavior. On some of the outcome measures, rational restructuring was comparably effective to behavior rehearsal. However, the findings suggest that a combination of the two is likely to be most effective. The clinical utility of rational restructuring as a way of facilitating assertive behavior has similarly been determined by Martorano, Nietzel, and Melnick (1977).

A study by Lent, Russell, and Zamostny (1981) found that cue-controlled desensitization was more effective than rational restructuring in the reduction of public speaking anxiety, However, comparable effectiveness of rational restructuring at the follow-up assessments suggests that the intervention period may have been too brief for the results to be manifested at posttesting. Some interesting post hoc findings by Casas (1975) suggest that rational restructuring may be particularly effective in the reduction of public speaking anxiety for those individuals who score high on a measure reflecting their excessive concern regarding the opinion of others.

In a collaborative study conducted at both Stony Brook and Catholic University, Goldfried, Linehan, and Smith (1978) found rational restructuring to be an effective procedure in the reduction of test anxiety when compared to either a waiting list control or a treatment procedure involving only the imaginal exposure to test-taking situations. Although imaginal exposure was more effective than the waiting list control, the addition of the cognitive coping factor to the imaginal exposure in the rational restructuring procedure served to further enhance anxiety reduction. Similar findings were obtained by Osarchuk (1974), who also determined that rational restructuring was comparably effective as self-control desensitization and a combination of both rational restructuring and desensitization. Wise and Haynes (1983) found that although rational restructuring was more effective than a waiting list control condition in reducing test anxiety, it was no more effective than attentional training, in which individuals were taught to focus their attention on the test-taking task. When taken together with other related research in this area (see Goldfried, 1979), it appears that the *coping emphasis* inherent in rational restructuring may be the effective ingredient in the treatment of test anxiety, rather than the specific nature of the rational restructuring intervention itself.

Jenni and Wollersheim (1979) compared rational restructuring with a stress management training program based on relaxation training in the treatment of Type A behavior. Both conditions were found to be more effective in reducing state, but not trait anxiety when compared to a waiting list control. The two treatments were equally effective in reducing state and trait anxiety, but neither was able to lower cholesterol level or blood pressure. Rational restructuring, however, was more effective than stress management in lowering the Type A behavior in itself.

A case report by Hamberger and Lohr (1980) has illustrated the effective use of rational restructuring in the treatment of anger. In a controlled study on anger reduction that compared rational restructuring with coping relaxation, Hazeleus and Deffenbacher (1986) found the two to be equally effective and superior to a no-treatment control. However, the rational restructuring was more effective in the amelioration of other problems, particularly that of generalized anxiety.

Finally, a case report by Harvil (1984) has included rational restructuring as part of an intervention procedure for the successful treatment of bulimia. Because of the nature of this report, however, it is not possible to generalize these findings beyond the single case.

THERAPEUTIC PROCEDURE

Most forms of therapy are alike in that they provide the opportunity for clients to obtain a different perspective on problematic aspects of their lives. The goal of rational restructuring is not only to accomplish this objective but also to teach clients a procedure by which they may do this *for themselves*. In this regard, the goal of this therapeutic procedure may be viewed as providing individuals with coping skills

(Goldfried, 1980b), so that they may ultimately learn to function as their own therapists.

There are a variety of ways that the general principles underlying rational restructuring may be translated into therapeutic technique. Methods for assisting clients in obtaining a different perspective on themselves or their lives will vary depending upon one's particular theoretical orientation. As yet, we have no clear empirical support for the efficacy of any one particular procedure over another in achieving this goal.

As indicated above, rational restructuring was based on the work of Ellis, who has been a strong proponent for the need to change one's thinking as a way of altering maladaptive emotions and actions. Systematic rational restructuring was devised as an attempt to provide somewhat more structure to this type of therapeutic intervention and to place greater emphasis on the use of this procedure for providing individuals with personal coping skills. The clinical procedure of rational restructuring is much like that of self-control desensitization described in Chapter 5, except that clients use rational reevaluation instead of relaxation skills to cope with anxiety. This reevaluation process is designed to help them differentiate between a real threat in the environment and something that is erroneously perceived as being dangerous. What follows are clinical guidelines, together with illustrative transcripts, that describe the implementation of this procedure.

(1) Presenting the Assumption That Thoughts Mediate Emotions

The initial therapy goal is to help clients recognize that their thoughts, assumptions, expectations, and labels—however fleeting or automatic—can affect their emotional reaction to situations. Although there are instances in which clients can readily identify thoughts that lead to emotional reactions, the therapist should also emphasize that there may be other instances in which we may not literally "tell ourselves" things that elicit emotional reactions, particularly if these thoughts have been so well learned that they assume the status of an automatic and implicit construction of events. It is often helpful to emphasize to clients that they are reacting "as if" they were perceiving a particular situation in a given way. Inasmuch as the goal at this particular point is simply to help clients gain an appreciation of the assumption that the perception of events can have an influence on anxiety reactions, a detailed discussion of the nature of the specific thoughts that are mediating their anxiety would not be required.

The following illustrative transcript from Goldfried and Davison (1976) provides an example of how this initial step may be implemented. Also included in the transcript within brackets are the therapist's thoughts and decision-making processes.

Client: My primary difficulty is that I become very uptight when I have to speak in front of a group of people. I guess it's just my own inferiority complex.

Therapist: [*I don't want to get sidetracked at this point by talking about that conceptualization of his problem. I'll just try to finesse it and make a smooth transition to something else.*] I don't know if I would call it an inferiority complex but I do believe that people can, in a sense, bring on their own upset and anxiety in certain kinds of situations. When you're in a particular situation, your anxiety is often not the result of the situation itself, but rather the way in which you *interpret* the situation—what you tell yourself about the situation. For example, look at this pen. Does this pen make you nervous?

Client: No.

Therapist: Why not?

Client: It's just an object. It's just a pen.

Therapist: It can't hurt you?

Client: No.

Therapist: If, instead, I were holding a gun or knife, would that make you nervous?

Client: Yes.

Therapist: But a gun or knife is also just an object. Unlike a pen, however, a gun or a knife *can* actually hurt you. It's really not the object that creates emotional upset in people, but rather what you think about the object [*Hopefully, this Socratic-like dialogue will eventually bring him to the conclusion that self-statements can mediate emotional arousal.*] If you had never seen a gun or a knife, do you think you would be upset?

Client: Probably not.

Therapist: [*Now to move on to a more interpersonally relevant example, but not yet one that samples the present problem.*] Now this holds true for a number of other kinds of situations where emotional upset is caused by what a person tells himself about the situations. Take, for example, two people who are about the attend the same social gathering. Both of them may know exactly the same number of people at the party, but one person can be optimistic and relaxed about the situation, whereas the other one can be worried about how he will appear, and consequently very anxious. [*I'll try to get him to verbalize the basic assumption that attitude or perception is most important here.*] So, when these two people walk into the place where the party is given, are their emotional reactions at all associated with the physical arrangements at the party?

Client: No, obviously not.

Therapist: What determines their reactions, then?

Client: They obviously have different attitudes toward the party.

Therapist: Exactly, and their attitudes—the ways in which they approach the situation-greatly influence their emotional reactions.

Source: Goldfried & Davison. 1976, pp. 163–165.

As can be seen in the example given above, the therapist has described the significance of thoughts and its implications for emotions in a very general way, and has not yet dealt specifically with the client's problems. Inasmuch as an analysis of the thoughts that may be mediating the particular client's anxiety reaction is likely to be considerably more complicated, it is important that this particular phase be used merely to gain acceptance of the basic rationale underlying the intervention to come. As another helpful means of conveying the underlying rationale, self-help books such as those by Burns (1980, 1985) and Ellis and Harper (1975) may be usefully employed.

(2) Eliciting a Realistic Perspective From the Client

Rather than having the therapist attempt to convince clients that their anxiety-arousing assumptions are unrealistic, the goal here is to assist them in gaining this perspective on their own. One way in which this may be accomplished is by having the therapist play devil's advocate, so that the client's task is to convince the seemingly unrealistic therapist why his or her way of thinking does not make sense. The therapist may present these assumptions in extreme form, which not only can increase the likelihood that the client will disagree with them but also will make it easier for the client to offer reasons that this particular belief may be unrealistic (e.g., "If I am not loved and approved of by everyone for everything that I say and do, then this is proof that I am an unworthy person"). The therapist may note that this does not necessarily imply that the client is indeed this extreme in his or her viewpoint, but rather that this is a vehicle that can help one to gain a better perspective on certain assumptions. Thus the objective of the therapist is to have clients make the distinction between the thought that "it would be nice" if certain things happened in comparison to the hope that they "must" or "should" occur.

The rationale for the therapist playing devil's advocate is based on social psychological literature that suggests having individuals *themselves* offer arguments to refute a given point of view is more effective than having another person provide them with the alternative perspectives (Brehm & Cohen, 1962).

The particular beliefs that would be selected for inclusion in this exercise should be based on what the therapist judges to be the underlying assumptions mediating the client's anxiety reaction. In the case of anxiety associated with social situations, the belief that "Everyone must love and approve of me" is likely to underlie the fear of criticism and rejection. In anxiety associated with achievement-oriented situations, the concern about disapproval from others may operate, but in addition may involve the mediating assumption that "I must be perfect in everything I do." In making a decision as to which underlying assumption to work with, it is clear that a great deal depends on the therapist's clinical formulation of the case at hand.

The following is a clinical illustration of how the devil's advocate exercise may be implemented:

Therapist: I would like to do something with you. I'm going to describe a certain attitude or belief to you, and I'd like you to assume for a moment that I actually hold this belief. What I would like you to do is to offer me as many reasons as you can why it may be irrational or unreasonable for me to hold on to such a belief. OK?

Client: All right.

Therapist: Assume that I believe the following: Everybody must approve of me, and if this doesn't happen, it means that I am really a worthless person. What do you think of that?

Client: I don't think it makes much sense.

Therapist: [*We're off to a relatively good start. A certain percentage of clients—fortunately a small percentage—will initially acknowledge that the belief does not seem irrational to them. But now he has to be more specific.*] But why doesn't it make much sense?

Client: You really can't expect that people are going to do that.

Therapist: [*Naïvely*] Why not?

Client: It just seems unreasonable for you to expect that they would.

Therapist: [*We don't seem to be getting anywhere. I can prompt him indirectly by being a bit more extreme in my belief, hopefully making counter-arguments a bit more obvious.*] I feel that every single person that I run into during the course of the day is going to have to smile and say nice things to me. And if this doesn't happen, I really feel down.

Client: But the world is simply not set up that way. There may be people who don't react to you positively because of things that are going on with themselves.

Therapist: [*That's a good reason but it needs some elaboration.*] What other reasons could there be? I tend to think that everything is somehow caused by me.

Client: But that's ridiculous. It's possible that someone you meet may have had a bad night's sleep, or may have had an argument with his wife, and is in no mood to deal with you.

Therapist: [*I'll reinforce him by accepting this explanation, but then present another example of my irrationality.*] So you think that some of the day-to-day variations in the way people react to me can be due to things completely apart from my own adequacy?

Client: Of course.

Therapist: OK, that certainly is a possibility. But what about when someone is really disapproving of *me?* For example, a close friend may disagree with something I say. Now in that case, I usually feel that I am wrong, and I must be worthless for him to have disagreed with me.

Client: But you can't expect him to agree with everything you say.

Therapist: Why not?

Client: If you did, you would really be dishonest.

Therapist: But I feel that it is more important for me to get everyone to approve of me and like everything I say and do, than it is for me to really express the way I feel. In fact, I sometimes feel like a weather vane, shifting whichever way the wind might be blowing.

Client: But that's ridiculous! What happens to you as a person?

Therapist: [*He seems fairly strong on this point, so I think I'll back off a little.*] That seems to be a big problem with me; I often don't know who I am as a person. I seem to be so concerned about defining my own worth in terms of what everyone else's reactions are toward me. But how else can I think?

Client: Maybe you should consider how *you yourself* feel about certain things you do. Provided you're not really hurting anybody else, if you feel that what you are doing is right, perhaps you should be satisfied with that and realize that not everyone is going to agree.

Therapist: [*I'm satisfied that he sees the irrationality in that belief.*] That seems to make some sense. If I can only really accept it.

Client: You'll have to, because the other way is not at all reasonable.

Therapist: [*Stepping out of role*] OK. You seem to have a very good perspective on the rationality of that belief. Why don't we move on to another notion?

Source: Goldfried & Davison, 1976, pp. 166–168.

The objective of this particular phase of rational restructuring is not merely to have clients acknowledge that certain beliefs are unrealistic, but rather to generate as many specific reasons that they believe can account for the unrealistic nature of this assumption. Basically, the therapist's goal is to have the client generate such statements as "If other people disagree with you that doesn't mean they dislike you." As will be seen in a later step in the implementation of this treatment procedure, the statements that are generated by clients in trying to convince the therapist why certain assumptions are unrealistic may be personalized, so that they can use them for themselves. By changing references to "you" so that they are stated as "I," clients essentially have generated reasons that may be used as coping statements. At this point, however, the generation of more reality-based reasons is carried out on a more hypothetical basis.

(3) Identifying the Unrealistic Assumptions Mediating the Client's Anxiety

As a result of the previous step, clients often spontaneously recognize that certain implicit beliefs are relevant to their own anxiety reactions. If this is not the case, a more detailed explanation can be carried out, so that they become better aware of the specific assumptions that caused them to be anxious in various life situations. The particular situations reviewed during this phase may be arranged into a hierarchy that may be employed in the next phase of the therapy.

It is possible to analyze the things that clients are saying to themselves by examining the following two questions: (a) What is the likelihood that they are in fact correctly interpreting the situation? and (b) What are the ultimate implications of the way that they have labeled the situation? Consider a situation in which a woman becomes upset because a man to whom she was attracted does not accept an invitation to a party that she is giving. She might indicate that she is upset because she is interpreting his refusal as reflecting the fact that he does not like her. The realistic nature of this interpretation can be examined by other potential causes for his refusal of the invitation (e.g., other commitments he might have at the time). Thus in attempting to answer the first question that deals with the potential unrealistic nature of this woman's thoughts, other causal attributions for his reaction would need to be examined. In addressing the second question, one focuses on what may be considered a more "basic" assumption or schema. Thus the therapist may raise the question: "Let's suppose that he, in fact, *does not* like you, and this is the reason he refused the invitation. Why does this make you so upset? What are the other things that you may be implicitly thinking about his not liking you? What meaning do you attribute to this?" Further probing may be required (e.g., "Yes, but why should *that* upset you?") in order to get at the underlying schema that is driving her emotional reaction, such as the belief that she must be accepted and approved of by others.

A therapist will know that he or she has successfully implemented this particular phase when clients acknowledge that they recognize that certain assumptions—however implicit—are mediating their anxiety, but that merely being aware of this does not give them any guidelines on how they may change. Once clients have reached this point, they are ready for the next phase of the intervention.

(4) Helping Clients in Reevaluating Unrealistic Beliefs

The therapeutic work that has been outlined thus far is designed to help clients better understand how their evaluations of situations have been contributing to their anxiety, and to offer them some potential tools by which they may cope. However, simply being aware of the cause of one's anxiety does little to reduce it; what is needed is an active attempt at coping.

In helping clients to make use of rational restructuring as a means of coping with their anxiety, their emotional reaction must serve as a "signal" for them to stop and ask themselves: "What am I telling myself that may be unrealistic in this particular situation?" The therapeutic task is to assist them in identifying and then replacing this unrealistic evaluation with a more appropriate appraisal of the situation. Inasmuch as this often goes counter to their typical reaction when experiencing anxiety, it is rare for clients to immediately experience success in coping. Indeed, the coping process is initially difficult and tedious to implement, and can only be mastered with repeated practice.

This relearning process may be implemented in a number of different ways, including the use of imaginal rehearsal, attempts at application between sessions, work within group settings, and by means of procedural variations and therapeutic aids.

Imaginal rehearsal. Inasmuch as rational restructuring involves helping clients to think more realistically while they are actually in anxiety-producing situations, this relearning process may be implemented within the consultation session through imaginal rehearsal. As noted earlier, rational restructuring by means of imaginal presentation is similar to the self-control variation of systematic desensitization (see Chapter 5), in which clients are instructed to "remain in the situation" until they have successfully reduced their anxiety. In the case of desensitization, relaxation is used to cope; here cognitive reevaluation is employed.

Clients are asked to note how anxious they feel when imagining a particular situation, and then to identify what it is that they are saying to themselves that may be creating the upset. Clients are asked to "think aloud" during this process, so that the therapist may prompt them in their attempts at either ferreting out or reevaluating their perception of the event. Following the reevaluation process, they then note the extent to which their anxiety has decreased. The anxiety-arousing situations for which clients are provided with practice should represent concrete events that are likely to occur in their lives. These situations may be arranged in hierarchical fashion, with successful coping at one level determining progress to the next situation in the hierarchy. A more detailed discussion of selecting situations for imaginal rehearsal may be found in Goldfried and Davison (1976, 1994).

Inasmuch as the more realistic reevaluation of upsetting situations represents a relatively novel and complex thinking process, it is often helpful for the therapist to model the actual procedure. In the case of interpersonal anxiety, therapists can think aloud along the following lines:

I'm standing here at a party where I know relatively few people. Everybody seems to be talking in small groups, and I'm not feeling part of things. I'm starting to become tense. On a scale of 1 to 100% tension, I'm about at a level of 40. OK, what is it that I'm thinking that may be creating this anxiety? I think I'm worried that I won't do well in this situation. What do I mean by that? That I might not know what to say or might not come across well. And that would bother me because . . . because I would look foolish to these people. And that would bother me because . . . because they would think badly about me. And why does that upset me? That would upset me because . . . because that would mean that there is something wrong with me. Wait a minute. First of all, what are the chances that they think that of me? I don't know that they would actually think that I was inadequate or anything. At worst, they might think that I was a quiet person. Second of all, even if they did think badly of me, that doesn't necessarily mean that that's the way I am. I just don't show the best side of me in groups. I would still be me. Now that I think this way, I don't feel quite as anxious as I did, perhaps more at an anxiety level of about 20.

Even though the therapeutic guidelines are relatively straightforward, clients often experience difficulty in both ferreting out and reevaluating their evaluation of situations. Consequently, the therapist's clinical skill and sensitivity may be required, as illustrated in the following transcript:

Therapist: I'd like you to close your eyes now and imagine yourself in the following situation: You are sitting on stage in the auditorium, together with the other school board members. It's a few minutes before you have to get up and give your report to the people in the audience. Between 0 and 100 percent tension, tell me how nervous you feel.

Client: About 50.

Therapist: [*Now to get into his head.*] So I'm feeling fairly tense. Let me think. What might I be telling myself that's making me upset?

Client: I'm nervous about reading my report in front of all these people.

Therapist: But why does that bother me?

Client: Well, I don't know if I'm going to come across all right . . . .

Therapist: [*He seems to be having trouble. More prompting on my part may be needed than I originally anticipated.*] But why should that upset me? That upsets me because . . .

Client: . . . because I want to make a good impression.

Therapist: And if I don't . . .

Client: . . . well, I don't know. I don't want people to think that I'm incompetent. I guess I'm afraid that I'll lose the respect of the people who thought I knew what I was doing.

Therapist: [*He seems to be getting closer.*] But why should that make me so upset?

Client: I don't know. I guess it shouldn't. Maybe I'm being *overly* concerned about other people's reactions to me.

Therapist: How might I be overly concerned?

Client: I think this may be one of those situations where I have to please everybody, and there are an awful lot of people in the audience. Chances are I'm not going to get everybody's approval, and maybe that's upsetting me. I want everyone to think I'm doing a good job.

Therapist: Now let me think for a moment to see how rational that is.

Client: To begin with, I don't think it really is likely that I'm going to completely blow it. After all, I have prepared in advance, and have thought through what I want to say fairly clearly. I think I may be reacting as if I already have failed, even though it's very unlikely that I will.

Therapist: And even if I did mess up, how bad would that be?

Client: Well, I guess that really wouldn't be so terrible after all.

Therapist: [*I don't believe him for one moment. There is a definite hollow ring to his voice. He arrived at that conclusion much too quickly and presents it without much conviction.*] I say I don't think it'll upset me, but I don't really believe that.

Client: That's true. I would be upset if I failed. But actually, I really shouldn't be looking at this situation as being a failure.

Therapist: What would be a better way for me to look at the situation?

Client: Well, it's certainly not a do-or-die kind of thing. It's only a ridiculous committee report. A lot of the people in the audience know who I am and what I'm capable of doing. And even if I don't give a sterling performance, I don't think they're going to change their opinion of me on the basis of a five-minute presentation.

Therapist: But what if some of them do?

Client: Even if some of them do think differently of me, that doesn't mean that I *would* be different. I would still be me no matter what they thought. It's ridiculous of me to base my self-worth on what other people think.

Therapist: [*I think he's come around as much as he can. We can*

terminate this scene now.] With this new attitude toward
the situation, how do you feel in percentage of anxiety?

Client: Oh, about 25 percent.

Therapist: OK, let's talk a little about some of the thoughts you had
during that situation before trying it again.

Source: Goldfried & Davison, 1976, pp. 172–174.

As can be seen in the above transcript, the therapist plays an active role in the rational restructuring procedure. Just how active a role
depends on the extent to which the client is experiencing difficulty in
the use of the procedure. As the client becomes better able to identify
and reevaluate unrealistic interpretations of situations, the therapist
may gradually become less active and directive.

In using rational restructuring clinically, I have found that clients
may be assisted in uncovering their unrealistic assumptions by the use
of *incomplete sentences.* Thus the therapist may introduce such
thoughts as "If people noticed that I made a mistake it would bother
me because . . ." and "and *that* would bother me because. . . ." As
clients' interpretations of situations often reflect the *implicit* meaning
that they attribute to an event, the use of incomplete sentences can often help to clarify this latent meaning structure.

Between session applications. Clients are encouraged to
make use of the rational restructuring procedure in real-life settings
whenever they experience anxiety. They should be forewarned, however, that inasmuch as real-life situations do not occur in a hierarchical fashion, they may encounter situations with which they may have
difficulty in coping. They can be told, however, that even if they are
not successful in reducing anxiety, attempts to apply this procedure in
real life can nonetheless provide them with practice in developing the
set to cope. With increased practice, these coping attempts should be
expected to become more effective. Written records of their attempts
at coping can make use of a homework sheet consisting of a page with
five columns labeled as follows: description of situation, initial anxiety
level (0–100), unrealistic thoughts, realistic reevaluation, and subsequent anxiety level (0–100).

Application in group settings. Rational restructuring may
readily be used within a group setting, a format within which its effec-

tiveness in treating test anxiety (Goldfried et al., 1978), interpersonal anxiety (Kanter & Goldfried, 1979), and anger (Hazeleus & Deffenbacher, 1986) has been studied. Not only is the group setting an economical way of treating a larger number of clients, but other members of the group may also serve as models for the successful implementation of the procedure. Depending on one's circumstances, the group implementation may vary. Thus, if the group is composed of clients with a common problem (e.g., social anxiety), a standardized hierarchy may be used. If the nature of the problem varies, or if for other reasons it is not possible to use a standardized hierarchy, each group member can have the situations most relevant to him or her written on index cards for individual use.

When rational restructuring is conducted in groups, the setting lends itself particularly well to the use of behavior rehearsal, especially in instances involving interpersonal anxiety. In dealing with such issues, coping (cognitively and behaviorally) with anxiety-producing situations may he simulated within the group itself. Anxiety in public speaking situations similarly may be most effectively implemented in group settings, where clients can learn to reevaluate their anxiety-arousing expectations while presenting actual practice speeches before fellow group members.

Variations and therapeutic aids.   Rational restructuring may be construed as facilitating an internal dialogue between two implicit sides of an individual—the realistic and unrealistic parts of a person. In light of this, the gestalt two-chair exercise can be used to more clearly underscore the nature of the dialogue. Thus the therapist can explain that the exercise involves taking what is internal and implicit and making it *external* and *explicit*. The clients' task is to dialogue with themselves, changing chairs each time they assume a different vantage point, with the therapist prompting as necessary. In using this procedure clinically, one often notices a greater amount of emotional arousal than with imaginal rehearsal, eliciting what might be construed as "hotter" cognition.

A therapeutic aid that many clients respond to favorably consists of bibliotherapy. Self-help books such as those written by Burns (1980, 1985) and Ellis and Harper (1975) not only illustrate how one's perception of situations leads to emotional upset, but also contain many case examples of how other people have been able to reevaluate their misperception of events.

APPLICATIONS OF RATIONAL RESTRUCTURING

Rational restructuring should be considered as an appropriate intervention procedure for various forms of anxiety that are believed to be mediated by the client's inappropriate appraisal of the situation. Particularly, various forms of social-evaluative anxiety are typically mediated by excessive concerns over the negative reactions of others. Thus within both private practice and clinic settings, rational restructuring would be most appropriate with cases of social anxiety and unassertiveness. In addition. it would be relevant in those instances of public speaking and test-taking anxiety that are believed to be related to the anticipated reactions of others. Although it also can be used as a procedure for reducing anger, available research has not demonstrated its superiority to the use of coping relaxation.

There is also clinical and research evidence to suggest that rational restructuring may be helpful when a client's problems stem from unrealistically high standards. Although individuals may be objectively competent in the way they deal with life events, they may nonetheless experience anxiety because they fall short of the expectations they hold for themselves. The preliminary work conducted on the use of rational restructuring for the treatment of Type A behavior (Jenni & Wollersheim, 1979) attests to the appropriateness of this intervention for such problems.

There is little research evidence available to suggest how individual client differences interact with the effectiveness of rational restructuring. In clinical practice, however, it is clear that rational restructuring is often most appropriately used together with a variety of other intervention procedures, depending upon the case at hand. Thus in cases of social anxiety where individuals also lack certain interpersonal skills, a combination of rational restructuring and behavioral rehearsal would be indicated. Similarly, there may be times when relaxation procedures should be used prior to the implementation of rational restructuring, particularly in cases when clients are experiencing high levels of anxiety that prevent them from identifying and reevaluating their misperceptions of situations.

Rational restructuring is unlikely to make much impact on individuals manifesting a formal thought disorder, such as paranoid schizophrenics. The strong biochemical component involved in such disorders calls more for pharmacotherapy than for a procedure like rational restructuring. In applying rational restructuring with populations where it *is* deemed appropriate, the therapist should be careful not to use it as a purely intellectual exercise. The client needs to learn to make use of these reevaluation skills to cope with anxiety, and consequently should experience a certain level of anxiety when the method is being employed.

One final point may be made before concluding. Rational restructuring can be construed as a treatment to use in those cases of anxiety when direct exposure to the client's feared consequences are typically not possible, such as when they involve what other people think and the implications that such evaluations have for the client. In many respects, rational restructuring may be seen as a *cognitively-implemented exposure procedure*, in the sense that clients are provided with the opportunity to consider the possible impact they may have on others and then to reevaluate the consequences of this in light of their contemporary life situation.

SUMMARY

This chapter has outlined the theoretical assumptions and research base for rational restructuring, a cognitive-behavioral intervention procedure that may be used for the reduction of certain anxiety-related disorders. Specifically applicable to various forms of social-evaluative anxiety, such as social anxiety, unassertiveness, public speaking, and test-taking anxiety, the goal of rational restructuring is to help clients to learn to obtain a more realistic perspective on themselves and their relationships with others. In the most general sense, rational restructuring may be construed as a procedure for teaching clients the use of a coping skill. Intervention procedures within the consultation session were described and illustrated, and suggestions were offered for the application of this coping skill in the client's life.

7

On the Facilitation of
Self-Efficacy

Numerous personality theorists have emphasized the importance of individuals having a feeling of control over significant events in their lives, describing this sense of competence, mastery, or effectance as a central motivator of human behavior (e.g., Rotter, 1954; Seligman, 1975; White, 1959). Although it is not always made an explicitly central goal, it appears that a wide variety of psychotherapies similarly make use of the concept of mastery. Among earlier writers, Adler (1930) in particular emphasized the need to experience control over one's environment in order to achieve a state of psychological well-being. Glasser's (1965) reality therapy has similarly focused on the importance of patients assuming responsibility for their own choices. Cognitive therapy, such as that outlined by Beck (1967, 1976), deals with depressed clients' views of themselves as helpless beings by providing them with graded tasks so that successes are experienced. More semantic therapies such as Ellis's (1962) rational-emotive therapy and Frankl's (1965) logotherapy attempt to teach clients control over their beliefs and attitudes about external events. Finally, cognitive-behavior therapy in general may be viewed as training in coping skills (Goldfried, 1980b), the end result of which is an increased sense of personal mastery.

There is considerable evidence from both basic and applied research that points to a variety of beneficial effects arising from perceived internal control. Much of the laboratory work has been reviewed by Lefcourt (1976) and by Phares (1976). For example, it has been shown that physiological and subjective reactions to aversive events (e.g. shock) are lessened under conditions of perceived control

over the events (Geer, Davison, & Gatchel, 1970), even if the subject
never used this potential control (Glass, Singer, & Friedman, 1969). In
the area of outcome research, Davison, Tsujimoto, and Glaros (1973)
found that when subjects were told that the drug used in the treatment of their insomnia was a placebo, the maintenance of improvement was enhanced. Somewhat similar results were reported by
Chambliss and Murray (1979) with smoking reduction, where it was
found that only clients whose locus of control was internal benefited
from this communication. Goldfried and Trier (1974) report that
training subjects in relaxation as a coping skill resulted in the reduction of speech anxiety, whereas training subjects in relaxation that was
construed as an automatic inhibitor of anxiety did not. Perhaps some
of the most remarkable evidence for the importance of perceived control comes from a study by Langer and Rodin (1976), which revealed
that nursing home residents who were given a communication stress-
ing their responsibilities and choices, and who were provided with a
house plant to look after, were later rated as happier, more active, and
more alert than residents for whom it was emphasized that these responsibilities belonged to the staff. In a follow-up study (Rodin &
Langer, 1977), not only did these differences continue, but the former
group actually lived longer.

The notion of perceived control or mastery has provided the basis
for Bandura's (1977) self-efficacy theory. Although having some similarities to earlier conceptualizations, self-efficacy theory is more detailed in the sense that it specifies the nature of the situation and response but at the same time is integrative by virtue of its broad scope
of applicability. The primary purpose of this chapter is to outline procedural guidelines that may be useful in facilitating self-efficacy
within the clinical context. Following a brief description of the current theoretical and research status of self-efficacy theory, we move on
to a more detailed discussion of what therapists can actually do to assist clients in cognitively processing learning experiences that bear on
their personal self-efficacy. These guidelines follow from basic theory
and research in social and cognitive psychology, as well as from clinical experience in utilizing cognitive-behavioral procedures. Included
with these guidelines are some illustrative clinical transcripts. Finally,
we touch upon some of the clinically related research questions that
need to be addressed on this general topic.

OVERVIEW OF SELF-EFFICACY THEORY

The basic assumption associated with Bandura's (1977) self-efficacy theory is that "psychological procedures, whatever their form, serve as ways of creating and strengthening expectations of personal efficacy." A particularly innovative aspect of Bandura's presentations is the distinction between *outcome expectancies*, referring to "a person's estimate that a given behavior will lead to certain outcomes," and *efficacy expectancies*, defined as "the conviction that one can successfully execute the behavior required to produce the outcomes." Bandura's primary emphasis is on efficacy expectancies, which are believed to determine people's choice of behavioral settings and activities, the amount of effort they will expend, and how long they will persist in the face of obstacles. Thus, a man who feels incompetent in heterosocial situations may avoid parties; if he finds himself at one, he may not make attempts to converse with women; if he does, he will soon desist if they do not give a very clear indication of interest. In addition to influencing how individuals will behave, efficacy expectancies are also viewed as affecting one's thought processes and emotional reactions.

Unlike broader trait conceptions such as locus of control, self-efficacy theory refers to expectancies about very specific interactions with one's environment. Further, efficacy expectations are said to vary on several dimensions that influence actual performance. First, they may differ in magnitude, as in which tasks in a hierarchy one can successfully handle. Secondly, they may differ in strength, or the extent to which people believe they can perform the behavior. Finally, they may differ in generality or the degree to which similar expectancies are held for behaviors in other situational contexts.

Efficacy expectancies can be based on different sources of information, and the various modes of therapy differ in the particular sources of information that they emphasize (Bandura, 1977). According to Bandura, performance accomplishments (such as those resulting from *in vivo* desensitization, direct exposure, participant modeling, etc.) are the most dependable and therefore the most heavily weighted sources of efficacy information. This is due to the person's first hand observation of improved performance and to their perceived development of coping skills with which to meet future situations. While observation of others can affect a client's perceived efficacy, this source of information is much less dependable than one's own experience. Verbal persuasion, while it may make some impact, also tends to lead to weaker changes in expectancies. Finally, emotional arousal may affect efficacy expectancies, since many people have learned that their performance deteriorates under conditions of high arousal.

Although Bandura has associated various treatment methods with each of these different sources of efficacy information, it seems plausible that most treatments provide information from more than one source. For example, while relaxation and desensitization procedures may be construed as reducing emotional arousal, they can also provide information to clients about their performance accomplishments, i.e., that they are learning a behavioral skill that can be used to overcome anxiety on future occasions (cf. Goldfried, 1980b). Similarly, problem-solving training provides clients with performance feedback and also, by focusing on realistic outcomes and their likelihoods, may reduce the emotional arousal generated by catastrophizing and employing vague generalizations. And while cognitive restructuring may primarily seem to employ verbal persuasion, clinical experience suggests that cognitive changes are not fully made, or do not endure, unless backed up by attention to successful performances on those tasks that have been attempted as a result of the cognitive therapy.

STATUS OF SELF-EFFICACY THEORY

Empirical evidence has appeared in support of self-efficacy theory. In a treatment study with snake phobics, Bandura, Adams, and Beyer (1977) found that efficacy expectancies and actual performance accomplishments were higher for those subjects treated by participant modeling than for those given modeling alone, which in turn exceeded the expectancies and performance of those in the no-treatment group. This finding supports the assumption that performance accomplishments provide the most dependable information for efficacy expectancies. Further, subjects' efficacy expectancies were more predictive of posttest performance than was their past behavior (i.e., terminal therapy performance), thereby supporting the utility of the efficacy construct. Bandura and Adams (1977) reported that completely desensitized snake phobics had varying levels of self-efficacy, presumably due to different past experiences and/or cognitive appraisals. The self-efficacy ratings, however, were again highly predictive of their ability to approach a snake. In a second study, Bandura and Adams found expectancies and performance to rise closely together during the course of participant modeling, where, again, expectancies were a better predictor than past behavior. Although the original work in this area began with phobics, subsequent research on self-efficacy has been extended to such other areas as achievement behavior (Bandura & Schunk, 1980; Brown & Inouye, 1978), assertiveness (Kazdin, 1979), smoking cessation (Candiotte & Lichtenstein, 1980), physical stamina (Weinberg, Gould, & Jackson, 1979), and recovery from heart attack (Ewart, Taylor, & DeBusk, 1980).

Self-efficacy theory has not gone without criticism, nor have the data obtained in its support. A number of these critiques and a lengthy reply by Bandura appeared in special issue of *Advances in Behavior Research and Therapy*, edited by Rachman (1978). While it goes beyond the scope of this chapter to discuss any of these issues in detail, we might note that it was argued (Borkovec, 1978; Eysenck, 1978) that self-efficacy expectancies are simply epiphenomena that only reflect behavior change, and are in no sense its cause. For example, anxiety reduction in this view is said to be due entirely to unreinforced exposure to fearful stimuli. Bandura (1978) notes, however, that exposure alone cannot predict performance nearly as well as can expectancies. In reply to the related argument that not enough attention is given to conditioned anxiety (Borkovec, 1978; Eysenck, 1978; Lang, 1978; Wolpe, 1978), Bandura (1978) maintains that it is primarily perceived inefficacy that leads to anxiety, i.e., that anxiety is reactive, not conditioned. This viewpoint is very similar to that proposed by Lazarus and Launier (1978), who argue that the perception of the situation as being stressful is, in part, a function of the individual's ability to cope with that situation.

Quite apart from these criticisms of self-efficacy theory, it nonetheless seems to possess a number of advantages as a conceptualization of behavior change, some of which have been noted by Wilson (1978). It is a broad and integrative theory, seeking to explain a large body of data, articulating particularly well with the learned helplessness theory of depression (Abramson, Seligman, & Teasdale, 1978), and such cognitive methods as those outlined by Beck (1976). The theory is testable, since expectancies are measured independently of performance.

Further, it proposes specific expectancies, not global traitlike measures. Behavior therapists, ironically enough, have typically measured expectancies in a much more global way than they have measured overt behavior (see Rosenthal, 1978), and Bandura's work can offer us guidelines for future work on cognitive-behavioral assessment. Finally, apart from the theoretical concerns of whether or not self-efficacy expectancies are epiphenomena only resulting from actual behavior change, they may nonetheless provide us with a useful *clinical index* of the extent to which certain learning experiences have been cognitively processed by clients.

GUIDELINES FOR PROCESSING SUCCESS EXPERIENCES

A facet of self-efficacy theory that is particularly important in discussing clinical guidelines is the cognitive processing of information that could potentially affect a client's efficacy expectations. Indeed, it is not at all uncommon to observe clients who have encountered success experiences in certain areas of their lives but who fail to benefit from such events because of their tendency to overlook or otherwise ignore such experiences. Bandura (1977) has noted that information about personal efficacy can be either enhanced or attenuated by a number of cognitive factors. For example, performance-based information may be evaluated according to the attributed cause of the success or failure. Attributions for success that are external, specific, and unstable will lead to lower efficacy expectancies than internal, global, stable attributions for success. The reverse holds for failure attributions. These attributional styles have been found to be related to depression (Seligman, Abramson, Semmel, & von Baeyer, 1979), test anxiety (Metalsky & Abramson, 1981), and social anxiety (Sutton-Simon & Goldfried, 1982). Information that is vicariously derived by observing a model will also be differentially weighted according to factors such as perceived model characteristics (e.g., mastery or coping model, similarity to the observer) and situational factors (e.g., task difficulty, diversity of modeled attainments). Verbal persuasion information may be modified by perceived characteristics of the persuader, such as credibility, prestige, apparent expertise, and so forth. Emotional arousal information may be apprised as due to one's own inadequacy or to situational factors.

In each of these cases a judgment of personal efficacy is being made, partly on the basis of situational information, but also on the basis of individuals' generalized perceptions or schemas about themselves, other people, and the world (Metalsky & Abramson, 1981). Research in cognitive psychology by Tversky and Kahnemann (1974) has demonstrated that individuals tend to overlook objectively available evidence if this information is not representative of their more general theory of how things should be. In considering the general topic of human judgment and decision making, Einhorn and Hogarth (1978) present a model for why individuals tend to retain confidence in their inaccurate judgments, even in the face of potentially corrective experiences. They suggest that three factors may be operating: (a) Individuals may not search out and use evidence that disconfirms their expectations; (b) people may not be aware of environmental factors that may serve to constrain the occurrence of certain outcomes; and (c) one's memory may not adequately encode, store, and retrieve the relevant outcome information.

Work in social psychology (e.g., Ross, 1977) similarly indicates that in cases of conflict between generalized beliefs and situational information, people tend to rely more heavily on their beliefs, ignoring conflicting information. Having implications for self-efficacy is the finding that experimentally induced self-perceptions will persevere even when the evidence on which they have been based has been discredited (Ross, Lepper, & Hubbard, 1975).

Particularly relevant to the topic of self-efficacy expectancies is the research by Markus (1977) on self-schemas, which are described as "cognitive generalizations about the self, derived from past experience, that organize and guide the processing of the self-related information contained in an individual's social experience" (Markus, 1977, p. 63). Markus's findings reveal that having a well-developed self-schema for a particular behavioral domain (e.g., independence) facilitates judgments about the self in that domain, permits easier retrieval of confirming evidence, makes the individual more resistant to counterschematic information, and provides a basis for stronger predictions about future behavior than does having a less well-developed self-schema for that domain. This work suggests that efficacy expectancies for a behavior pattern depend upon or reflect the nature of an individual's self-schema for that particular area of functioning.

Having briefly noted some of the situational and cognitive parameters that may influence efficacy expectancies, the question becomes one of what therapists are to do when confronted with the difficult task of assisting clients in cognitively benefiting from the information generated by their successful encounters with the environment. In considering clinical strategies for facilitating perceived self-efficacy, we are assuming that the therapist has already been successful in encouraging clients to engage in new behaviors, and that he or she continues to do so. The behavioral techniques and the therapeutic relationship skills that can facilitate this have been extensively described by others. We will therefore focus on the cognitive processing ("working through"?) of these experiences, where the job of the therapist becomes that of (a) aiding the client in discriminating between past and present behaviors; (b) helping the client to view changes from both an objective and a subjective vantage point; (c) helping the client to retrieve past success experiences; and (d) aligning the client's expectancies, anticipatory feelings, behaviors, objective consequences, and subsequent self-evaluations. Although we have listed these strategies in an order that makes sense conceptually, it should not be assumed that they are necessarily carried out in that sequence. Rather, they are employed continuously throughout the course of treatment. The ultimate objective of these strategies is to effect a lasting change in clients' self-schemas.

Discrimination Between Past and Present

As clients begin to respond more effectively in their life situation, however minimal or temporary such changes may be, a critical issue is how the therapist should respond when clients report these changes during the consultation session. In addition to any attempts to reinforce clients for their novel responses, it is also important that the therapist discuss these changes in light of clients' previous behavior patterns.

The reasons for using the past as a point of comparison for current changes are threefold. To begin with, the behavior change process is a gradual and at times erratic one, and clients frequently become discouraged when they still remain far from their eventual goal.

Moreover, their actual changes may be minimized by assuming the "yes-but" attitude of: "Yes, but I have so much more to do." If clients are encouraged to evaluate their current responses in light of how they might have handled similar situations in the past, they are in a better position to appreciate how far they have come.

A second reason for using past responses as an anchor point for evaluating current changes is that competence and self-efficacy are not general traits but rather are specific to certain kinds of situations. For example, although clients may make significant gains in their ability to assert themselves with strangers, they may nonetheless continue to have assertion difficulties in their relationships with close friends. Consequently, they may discount their changes by maintaining: "Yes, but I can't do that in these other situations." Comparing their new behavior patterns with those occurring in similar situations in the past allows them to focus in on those particular areas of their life where they indeed have changed.

Finally, many clients will minimize their changes by contrasting their behavior with that of others (e.g., "Yes, but I can't do it as well as some other people"). Inasmuch as the competitive tendency to compare oneself against others is reinforced by our culture (e.g., "winning" is highly valued and being "second-best" is frowned upon), it is not surprising that such social comparison occurs fairly often in many clients. Noting that someone else may be able to respond more effectively in certain situations is likely to undermine the client's sense of self-efficacy (cf. Weinberg et al., 1979).

The following illustrative transcript indicates how one may use clients' past behavior in helping them to gauge their progress:

Client: I was able to tell my boss that I didn't want to work late on Thursday. It worked out fine and I really felt that I handled the situation nicely.

Therapist: I'm glad to hear that. What was the situation and how did you handle it?

Client: It was pretty much the same as always. She asked me Thursday after lunch if I could stay late and finish up some work that had to be ready by end of the week. I told her that I really couldn't do it, because I had some things that I had to do after work.

Therapist: How did you say it?

Client: In a very matter-of-fact way. I really didn't feel annoyed, so it really wasn't all that hard for me.

Therapist: Sounds good. I think it would be important if we compared how you handled this particular situation with how you typically responded in the past.

Client: Oh, I handled this much better.

Therapist: It certainly seems so. What specifically might you have said in the past?

Client: I would have said "yes," and then felt real angry at myself for doing it.

Therapist: So when this situation occurred in the past, you wouldn't say what you really wanted to say, and then would have felt badly, whereas now you spoke up, and felt good about it.

Client: That's right. And you know something . . . it really worked out okay. I mean, she didn't get angry or anything, and I told her that if I wasn't able to finish the work by Friday, I would stay a little bit later. As it turned out, I got it done in plenty of time.

Adding on Objective Vantage Point to Client's Subjective Outlook

Related to the need for contrasting current success with previous failures to cope is the ability of clients to assume an objective, as well as a subjective, view of their abilities. A number of studies summarized by Jones and Nisbett (1971) found that the attribution of the causes of a given behavior pattern differs depending on whether one is a participant in a given act or whether one is an observer. Typically, participants attribute the causes of their behavior to external situations, whereas observers find causes within the participants themselves. While this body of research is typically cited to illustrate how observers are more likely to make erroneous, traitlike conclusions about the causes of human behavior, and participants are more attuned to situational determinants, this objective-subjective distinction may also be seen as having relevance for self-efficacy expectations. That is, when interactions with the environment are viewed from a subjective vantage point, there is a built-in tendency for clients to see the causes of their novel success experiences as being due to something external to themselves, rather than to their own efforts. One may speculate that this phenomenon is, at least in part, "biological" in origin: Because people's eyes are situated within their heads, they are more likely to attend to the world around them than to themselves. Whether or not the participant's viewpoint is the more accurate one is of no importance here. Rather, we are concerned solely with a pragmatic issue. From the standpoint of enhancing self-efficacy, this attributional tendency is clearly countertherapeutic and warrants intervention by the therapist.

One of the characteristics that may indeed cut across diverse therapeutic orientations is that the therapist helps to bring about change by providing clients with an external, more objective perspective on their lives (Brady, Davison, Dewald, Egan, Fadiman, Frank, Gill, Hoffman, Kempler, Lazarus, Raimy, Rotter, & Strupp, 1980). In essence, the therapeutic goal is that of assisting clients to become not only participants in, but also observers of, their own lives. The external vantage point can be provided to clients in a number of ways, through the therapist's efforts (e.g., description of client behaviors, reflection, confrontation), by clients themselves (e.g., self-monitoring), or by feedback offered from significant others in the client's life. In addition to this more objective feedback, we have also found it most helpful clinically to juxtapose clients' objective perspective on someone else's ability to carry out a certain behavior pattern with their own distorted subjective view of themselves when they engage in the same behaviors. Wherever possible, therapists should allow clients to recognize by themselves the disparity between their subjective and an objective view of their behavior patterns. This may be seen in the following transcript, which is a continuation of the previous clinical interaction.

Client: I just feel that I'm always being taken advantage of, and get caught up in things that I really dislike.
Therapist: Such as?
Client: Like at work, I always seem to end up with the dirty work. When I look at other people, they don't seem to have the same problems. Like Lisa, for example . . . she handles herself much better than I ever can.
Therapist: What can she do that you can't?

Client: Well, she's not overburdened the way I am. She doesn't let other people take advantage of her.

Therapist: Can you give me some examples?

Client: It the boss comes in and there's extra work to be done, and she feels she's too busy with what she has to do, she's able to say something about it. I always go along with it.

Therapist: So like Lisa, you'd like to be better able to refuse to do extra work when it's inconvenient for you.

Client: Yes.

Therapist: Such as telling your boss that it's inconvenient for you to work late on a given day?

Client: (embarrassed) Uh . . . Well . . . But that was different.

Therapist: How so?

Client: (pause) I see what you're getting at. I guess it's just hard for me to see myself that way, But it's true; I *was* able to stand up for my rights in that situation.

Retrieval of Past Successes

In addition to engaging in new behavior patterns, and clearly recognizing that such changes reflect an improvement over past behavior, it is most important that clients "use" such success experiences to help guide their future actions. In order to raise self-efficacy expectancies, clients must not only behave in competent ways but must also view these behavior patterns as being part of their personal history. In addition, if performance has met with a positive outcome, this response-outcome link must also be fully recognized by clients and integrated into their self-schema. Unfortunately, many clients' personal histories consist more of failure than of success experiences, typically resulting in schemas that often provide built-in biases against new situational evidence. Inasmuch as such new information is more the exception than the rule — the existing rule having been based on numerous other experiences — the natural reaction is to minimize current perceptions and memories of positive experiences (Taylor & Crocker, 1981; Tversky & Kahnemann, 1974). This is consistent with clinical observations that increases in self-efficacy expectancies lag behind more objective performance accomplishments.

Despite the built-in bias against processing new information, schemas nonetheless are capable of being changed. For example, in addition to finding that self-perceptions tended to perseverate despite disconfirming evidence, Ross et al. (1975) observed that such distortions could be corrected by discussing with subjects the processes believed to be maintaining the perseveration. Within the clinical context, not only can one discuss this tendency to overlook new experiences, but it is also important to circumvent these biases by having clients self-monitor their successful coping efforts. By keeping such records, clients then have the potential of a readily available and objective reminder of their successes, which can also be used in helping to instigate future coping attempts. This should be supplemented by the therapist's periodic reminders of these effective responses, and conceptualized as comprising the beginnings of a totally new behavior pattern. While it is difficult to provide any hard-and-fast rules as to how long this deliberate process of retrieving past successes needs to be emphasized, clinical experience suggests that a "critical mass" of successful past attempts at coping need to be accumulated, providing, as it were, a turning point in the client's life. The exact number of such events differs widely from client to client, leaving this an important and as yet untouched area for future process research in behavior therapy.

The following transcript briefly illustrates a clinical interaction dealing with the retrieval of past success.

Therapist: Because you've had difficulty in asserting yourself for so long in the past, it's sometimes hard to keep in mind the changes that have been happening to you.

Client: I know. And it feels kind of different, almost as if it's not me that's doing it.

Therapist: That's certainly a natural part of the change process, which will probably continue until you start to build up more of a backlog of positive experiences. With each new situation you handle well, it should get a little easier. As a way of helping you to change, it's also important for you to remember the successes you have had.

Client: I do think of them sometimes.

Therapist: That's good, because there *is* a natural tendency to think of the more typical way you've reacted in the past — which is to *not* assert yourself — and that's why it's so important for you to really focus in on what seems to be a new pattern of handling situations on your part.

Client: Yes.

Therapist: In fact, when you think about your past successes, it can often help you to continue along those lines in the future. For example, when you finally speak to that friend of yours who is always showing up late, you might keep in mind successful instances of assertiveness you've experienced in the past. Before speaking to this friend, you might say to yourself something like: "I was able to say what was on my mind in these past situations, and I can do the same here as well." It doesn't have to be in those exact words; any way that you can remind yourself of past successes will help you in new situations where you want to stand up for your rights.

Aligning Expectancies, Anticipatory Feelings, Behaviors, Objective Consequences, and Self-Evaluation

In discussing the more general issue of negative self-concept, Goldfried and Davison (1976; 1994) suggest that the three interrelated parameters associated with adverse attitudes toward oneself involve the possibility that (a) clients' behavior patterns may be less than adequate, either because of skill deficits or response inhibitions; (b) clients' standards for self-evaluation may be unrealistically high; and/or (c) clients may be unaware of the impact they are making on their environment. In many clinical instances where clients report on their inadequate self-efficacy expectations, all three factors may be operating. As they begin to develop more effective behavior patterns, it is the job of the therapist to assist them in using this information to update their image of themselves. Stated in the language of cognitive psychology, the therapist focuses on events that might be "episodic" in nature, and assists clients in incorporating this event into a realigned "semantic memory" structure or schema (cf. Tulving, 1972).

As noted earlier, self-efficacy expectancies often lag behind behavior change. What one often encounters clinically are inconsistencies among the clients' expectations for success in a given situation, their anticipatory feelings prior to action, the response itself, the objective consequences, and their subsequent self-evaluation. In realigning the entire sequence of expectancies, feelings, action, consequences, and self-evaluation so that each phase is more consistent with the others, we have found it particularly important to deal with the subjective and experiential aspects reported by clients, as these are often most salient to them and indeed often constitute the cue to which they are reacting. For example, although emotional arousal may have been associated with ineffective performance in the past, there may come a time in the process of changing where clients end up functioning adequately even though they experience an initial period of emotional upset. In such instances, clients have available to them two conflicting sources of efficacy information—emotion and behavior—and it is important for the therapist to emphasize that although the emotional arousal may have been salient, it did not reliably predict effective performance in their recent past. Instead, clients would do well to focus on their *past success* when entering new, but similar situations. How this may be done clinically is perhaps best illustrated with the following example.

Therapist: Immediately before you told your boss that you couldn't work late that evening, what thoughts ran through your head?

Client: I don't know, it all happened so fast. I didn't want to stay late, but I was afraid to say anything about it.

Therapist: And some of your fears were . . . ?

Client: I was afraid my boss would get angry with me, that she would think I was not interested in my job. I didn't think that she would fire me or anything like that, but rather that she'd be annoyed at me.

Therapist: And despite these thoughts, you nonetheless decided to say something. What did you say to yourself that helped you to do that?

Client: That I worked hard all day, and that I really had other things to do.

Therapist: But these are thoughts you've had in past instances, where you *didn't* assert yourself. What did you think differently this time?

Client: Well, I had a fleeting thought that maybe I was being unrealistic. I also thought that I no longer wanted to always go along with what other people want, especially when it's not good for me.

Therapist: And what were your feelings right before you said anything?

Client: I was scared and nervous, but I spoke up anyway.

Therapist: And your response itself?

Client: It was straightforward and very matter-of-fact, even though inside I was shaking in my boots.

Therapist: And your boss's response?

Client: It wasn't really bad at all. In fact, she was even a little bit apologetic about having asked me. As I mentioned to you earlier, everything worked out okay anyway.

Therapist: Right. And how did you feel after it was all over?

Client: Well, I was certainly relieved. Nothing terrible happened; in fact, it turned out just fine.

Therapist: And how did you feel about *yourself?*

Client: Okay, I guess.

Therapist: You don't sound all that positive about this experience. If you had to evaluate yourself on a one to five scale, with five being most satisfied with yourself and one being least, how would you rate yourself?

Client: (pause): About a three.

Therapist: What would you have needed to do differently to have given yourself a five?

Client: (pause) I guess I would give myself a five if I didn't have this problem to begin with!

Therapist: But if we focus in on how you felt about your response in *this particular situation*, what would you have to do differently to give yourself a five?

Client: (pause) I don't know that I really could have done anything *any* differently. I guess it's just difficult for me to fully accept the fact that I handled it well. It's difficult for me to see myself in that way.

Therapist: I can understand that. But aren't you being overly harsh on yourself? At least in that situation?

Client: When you put it that way, I guess I am. I guess I did handle that situation fairly well.

Therapist: I think it's important for you to be real clear about what went on and how you handled it. If we step back and look at what went on, we have the following: You started off by being reluctant to say anything, for fear that something negative would happen. You were nervous, but still were able to talk yourself into speaking up. What you said certainly sounded appropriate, and was well received by your boss. The payoff was good, in that things turned out well.

Client: Right.

Therapist: There is a second payoff that you need to recognize as well, and that is that you have every right to feel good about yourself in that situation.

Client: I see what you're saying.

Therapist: Although this is only one small instance, it nonetheless can provide you with a good turning point, or something that you can fall back on in the future. Next time you're in a situation where you're afraid that something negative will happen if you speak up, and you also feel yourself apprehensive about doing so, think back about how these very same feelings occurred in this situation, how you were able to overcome them, and how things worked out well. It will probably take a number of such instances before you start to feel more self-confident about your ability to stand up for your own rights, but if you continue as you have, there's every reason to believe you'll eventually get there.

A fairly common observation among practicing clinicians is that with repeated instances such as that illustrated above, clients report that "something is happening" to them. Mahoney (1974) has referred to this phenomenon as the "cognitive click," whereby clients begin to reconstruct the image they have of themselves and their abilities. As they continue to accumulate more and more of such success experiences, processing this information within the therapy session helps them to realign their anticipatory thoughts and feelings with an appropriate self-evaluation of the outcome of their response. Eventually, a new behavior pattern, together with a greater sense of self-efficacy, begins to emerge.

SUGGESTED RESEARCH DIRECTIONS

While the primary purpose of this chapter has been to describe guidelines that may be used to enhance a client's self-efficacy expectations, our consideration of the concept of self-efficacy within the clinical context nonetheless raises some important research questions. Starting as a framework for studying snake phobics, self-efficacy theory provides a useful model for investigating other areas of functioning, such as the study of assertion, achievement behavior, interpersonal skills, self-regulation of addictive behaviors, self-care among the elderly, sexual problems, depression, as well as the whole gamut of phobic conditions. A relevant and interesting counterpoint to these problems involving *low* efficacy expectancies is the Type A personality, whose behavior pattern may be seen as reflecting efficacy expectancies that are *unrealistically high* across a wide range of situations (cf. Glass, 1977).

A particularly attractive feature of self-efficacy theory is that it takes into consideration individuals' cognitive processing of their learning experiences. It is probably because self-efficacy expectations are an end product of such intervening cognitive processes that they predict future behavior more accurately than does an objective account of the learning experience itself. These cognitive factors are an especially important set of parameters for future investigation.

As noted in earlier chapters, the notion of schema has assumed a central place in experimental cognitive psychology, where it has been used to explain the individual's contribution in the construction of perceptions and the distortions of memories (Bower, 1978; Neisser, 1976). Like Beck (1967, 1976), we suggest that this construct can similarly be useful in understanding the perception of and reaction to one's own behavior, interpersonal situations, and other clinically relevant stimuli, and may be particularly influential in determining how efficacy information is processed. This is well illustrated by Garber and Hollon's (1980) findings that in a skill task, depressed subjects showed smaller expectancy changes following success or failure than did nondepressed subjects, despite the fact that the two groups did not differ when estimating the probability of a model's future success. Thus, in spite of informational feedback, depressed subjects seemed to have extremely stable schemas concerning their own performance.

Suggesting that the schema construct is important in understanding self efficacy immediately raises a number of questions: How can various levels of clinically relevant schemas be directly assessed (cf. Chapter 4 and Landau & Goldfried, 1981)? How do schemas of various clinical groups differ from one another and from normals? Exactly how does schematic information interact with situational information to produce expectancies? What kinds of heuristics do people use in predicting their own behavior, and how do these differ from the rules employed in estimating how others will behave?

In addition to questions concerning the cognitive structures and processes underlying efficacy expectancies, research needs to address the parametric considerations associated with the types of therapist and client behaviors that may be useful in facilitating self-efficacy. Included among these parameters are the number of successful performances; the amount of self-monitoring or therapist reminders of such success; the degree to which these successes are actively compared with past failures; the extent to which clients compare their abilities to those of others; and the tendency to attribute success experiences to one's own efforts. These issues lend themselves particularly well to investigation through therapy process research, whereby therapists' behaviors can be monitored along with the ongoing changes in clients' emotional, cognitive, and behavioral functioning. Although there exists basic research in cognitive psychology on how schemas interrelate with cognitive processes, behavior, and emotion, there is little or nothing in the field that deals with the question of how schemas may be altered (Taylor & Crocker, 1981). It is our contention that researchers in cognitive psychology may be able to generate useful hypotheses about changing schemas from the experience of clinicians involved in facilitating self-efficacy expectations, and that the findings of any research derived in this way can in turn be fed back to help us enhance our clinical effectiveness.

SUMMARY

This chapter began by briefly considering the current theoretical and research status of self-efficacy theory, suggesting that self-efficacy expectations may provide us with a useful index of the extent to which certain learning experiences have been cognitively processed. Moreover, self-efficacy theory leads us in the direction of considering how individuals may actually go about encoding, storing, and retrieving corrective experiences, so as to alter self-efficacy expectations. The chapter discussed and illustrated procedural guidelines that may be useful in facilitating cognitive processing of efficacy information, whereby the role of the therapist becomes that of (a) aiding the client in discriminating between past and present behaviors; (b) helping the client to view changes from both an objective and a subjective vantage point; (c) helping the client to retrieve past success experiences; and (d) aligning the client's expectancies, anticipatory feelings, behaviors, objective consequences, and subsequent self-evaluations. The ultimate objective of these therapeutic strategies is to effect a lasting change in clients' self-schemas. Some of the clinically related research questions that need to be addressed have also been noted.

Part IV

EXPANDING THE SCOPE OF COGNITIVE-BEHAVIOR THERAPY

By their very nature, scientific fields are basically unstable social systems. As Parsons (1951) has pointed out:

> There is always the possibility that someone will make a new discovery. This may be merely a specific addition to knowledge of fact, in which case it will simply be fitted in with the rest in its proper place. But it may be something which necessitates the *reorganization* to a greater or lesser degree of the systematized body of knowledge. (p. 336)

Despite the fact that change is the avowed goal of any advancing field, there exists an essential tension between this hope for change and the need to maintain a status quo. In the case of psychotherapy in general, there clearly exist those who continue to practice the way they learned in their original training, despite advances that have occurred over the years.

In the relatively short period of time that behavior therapy has existed as a viable alternative to other orientations, it has made impressively rapid advances. Although many of the behavioral intervention methods have withstood the test of time, the practice of cognitive-behavior therapy in the 1990s is nonetheless different from what is was three decades earlier (Goldfried & Davison, 1994). In our original publication of *Clinical Behavior Therapy* in 1976, Davison and I commented on the past and future evolution of behavior therapy, suggesting:

> Behavior therapy is entering a new phase. We believe current and future developments will not only reflect a more sophisticated cognizance

117

of clinical activity, but will at the same time make the field more palatable to those hitherto put off by some of the narrow conceptualizations and polemics that marked the beginnings of behavior therapy. (Goldfried & Davison, 1976, p. 17)

Having its roots in experimental psychology, the growth and maturity of behavior therapy has been strongly influenced by basic and applied research findings. Less obvious, but nonetheless a very real force in the evolution of behavior therapy, have been the influences associated with attempts to apply behavioral procedures clinically. Much has been written about the gap between theory and research on the one hand, and actual clinical applications on the other. Although we may lament the discrepancies that exist between these two separate approaches to behavior therapy, the very fact that *each* of these separate vantage points has influenced the development of behavior therapy reflects a check and balance that is unique to therapy orientations.

Chapter 8 deals with the question of whether or not the growth of psychotherapy integration represents a mid-life crisis for cognitive-behavior therapy. Inasmuch as I have been personally involved in cognitive-behavioral research, training, and practice since the 1960s, the professional odyssey that I have experienced over these years is used to illustrate some of the changes that have been occurring in behavior therapy itself. The fact that my colleagues and I were not doing what the textbooks — including our own — said we should be doing is less of an indictment of cognitive-behavior therapy than an indication of its growth and evolution. To be on the growing edge of a discipline in no way negates its well-established body of knowledge, but rather openly admits that more needs to be done. Behavior therapy's period of self-examination is clearly a reflection of its strength, not weakness.

Chapter 9 provides a transcript of an interview by Windy Dryden, in which the focus was on dilemmas experienced by therapists in the course of their practice. The dilemma related in this chapter involves the case of a depressed man whom I was treating with assertiveness training. The goal of the therapy was to counteract his general level of passivity and dependence, hoping thereby to provide him with a greater sense of self-direction. Although the client originally agreed to the treatment plan, he was resistant throughout the early phases of therapy. It soon became apparent that this resistance was a form of passive-aggressiveness, reflecting the general interactional pattern he had with others in his life. In shifting my focus to our therapeutic interaction, I had to rationalize to myself that I was doing *"in vivo"* work, rather than analyzing the "transference." There currently seems to be less of a need for such a rationalization, as numerous other behavioral writers have strongly emphasized the need to focus on the therapist-client interaction as an essential component of a behavioral intervention (e.g., Arnkoff, 1983; Kohlenberg & Tsai, 1991; Linehan, 1993).

Acknowledging the contribution that psychodynamic therapy may make to behavior therapy in the form of evaluating the therapist-client interaction, Chapter 10 suggests that cognitive-behavior therapy may benefit from aspects of the change process that are essential to other therapeutic orientations. Based on a paper written with Adele Hayes, this chapter argues that uncovering the early origins of affect-laden schemas and relating them to current levels of functioning might be a useful addition to cognitive-behavioral interventions. Moreover, the growing interest in the role of affect in the psychotherapeutic change process can lead behavior therapists to attend more to the potential contributions made by experiential therapists.

In Chapter 11, some of the paradoxical limitations associated with behavior therapy's strengths are discussed. Although the contribution of behavior therapy was to move the field of therapy in a number of new directions, many of which have paid off quite handsomely in increasing our clinical effectiveness, it has also carried with it certain limitations. Based on an article written in collaboration with Louis Castonguay, this chapter maintains that behavior therapy's fine-grained analysis of human functioning has carried with it the danger of overlooking more global patterns of behavior; the emphasis on technique has diverted our attention from dealing with more general principles of change; the use of an educational model for teaching coping skills has brought with it the risk of using an overly didactic approach in our interventions; underscoring the importance of clients' current life in the real world has caused us to overlook what is happening in the therapeutic interaction itself; the efforts put into carrying out an impressive array of outcome research has diverted our attention from studying the therapy process; and our focus on devising methods for symptom reduction has kept us from developing and applying procedures that deal with clients' problematic interpersonal relations.

8

Psychotherapy Integration: A Mid-Life Crisis for Behavior Therapy?

In 1982, Kendall provided an Eriksonian developmental analysis of behavior therapy. He pointed out that through industry and hard work, behavior therapy finally reached an independent identity, and having done so — despite its chronological youth — was now in a better position to become intimate with other orientations.

When compared with other therapeutic orientations, behavior therapy has always been somewhat precocious. Born of creative minds and nurtured within both academic and clinical settings, behavior therapy quickly emerged as a protégé within the therapeutic community. Indeed, although still relatively young in years, it seems to be showing some signs of a mid-life crisis, asking such questions as: How far have I come until now, and what have I accomplished? Where have I fallen short of my expectations? What now? Will it be more of the same, or do I need to do something different?

There is no question but that we have made extraordinary strides in the past two to three decades. These have included important contributions made for the treatment of a wide variety of problems in children, major breakthroughs in dealing with anxiety disorders, launching the field of behavioral medicine, providing a powerful impetus to outcome research on psychosocial interventions, and the encouragement of other orientations to specify their therapeutic procedures, so that they would be better amenable to empirical test.

In the process of making such important contributions, behavior

therapy *itself* has evolved and grown, a maturation that is nicely outlined in a chapter by Glass and Arnkoff (1992), appearing in
Freedheim's edited volume on the *History of Psychotherapy*. Starting
as "conditioning therapies," behavior therapy has broadened its scope
so as to include the important role of the therapeutic relationship, the
recognition of the significance that cognitive variables may play in the
maintenance and alteration of clinical problems, and the development of procedures for dealing with marital distress. My sense is that
we are beginning to extend the horizons of behavior therapy still further, this time moving into the somewhat dangerous territory that has
traditionally been occupied by other orientations (cf., Beck, Freeman,
& Associates, 1990; Goldfried, 1982; Lazarus, 1977; London, 1986;
Mahoney, 1991; Meichenbaum & Gilmore, 1984).

Some years ago, Friedling, Goldfried, and Stricker (1984) surveyed
the therapeutic activities of Ph.D.s who graduated from Stony Brook and
from Adelphi University. Stony Brook graduates were trained to be behavioral, and the Adelphi Ph.D.s were trained within a psychodynamic
orientation. We developed a questionnaire, worded in ordinary English
so as to avoid offending jargon, which reflected the clinical practices as
carried out from within each of the two separate schools. Because each
item was generated from a given orientation, it was possible to determine
the extent to which participants made use of procedures from an orientation other than their own. As a result of this survey, we found that approximately 78% of the psychodynamic items were used by both orientations,
as were 55% of the behavioral practices. Such points of commonality included therapists indicating that they focus on specific situations and the
patient's/client's problematic reactions to them; using their own personal
reactions to understand their patient's/client's problems; pointing out
any behavior on the part of the patient/client that seems to interfere with
the work of therapy; focusing on the extent to which patient's/client's beliefs are unrealistic or rational; discussing patient's/client's day-to-day,
between-session activities; and providing feedback on the patient's/cli-
ent's in-session way of relating.

Apparently, many of these clinical psychologists, once having left the
academic nest, were no longer doing what the textbooks indicated they
should. The question was, why? We found no relationship at all with experience—the number of years since obtaining their degrees. What we
did find, however, was that among behavior therapists, the likelihood of
using psychodynamic procedures was positively correlated with the per-

centage of adult clients they were seeing, and negatively correlated with the percentage of child cases that typically comprised their practice. Among psychodynamic therapists, a positive relationship was obtained between their using behavioral methods and the percentage of lower socioeconomic patients seen. Inasmuch as approximately half of the Stony Brook graduates went on to academic/research careers, we were able to compare them with the practitioners that were trained in the same program. Not surprisingly, we found a higher degree of eclectic interventions among practicing clinicians.

What these findings suggest is a point made by Dollard and Miller (1950) some years ago when they indicated that people will not change unless they are confronted with a "learning dilemma," in which their tried-and-true methods of dealing with the world no longer seem to be working. I would hasten to add that the nature of the change in response to this learning dilemma is extremely important. Unfortunately, some behavior therapists have become totally disillusioned with the limitations associated with some of our currently-available procedures, and end up by totally rejecting the behavioral orientation altogether (e.g., Mozer, 1979). There are others, myself included, who continue to maintain their identity as a behavior therapist, and respond to this clinical need to expand our effectiveness by considering what other orientations might have to offer.

MY OWN PROFESSIONAL MID-LIFE CRISIS

This leads to the topic of my *own* professional mid-life crisis. I have been affiliated with one of the centers of behavior therapy—Stony Brook—since its inception in the mid-1960s, where numerous doctoral and postdoctoral students have received their behavioral training. Indeed, many former (and current) Stony Brook students have made, and continue to make, important contributions to the development of behavior therapy.

In the 1960s, the issue of concern to behavior therapy was that of the role of cognition. I remember reading Breger and McGaugh's 1965 *Psychological Bulletin* article critiquing behavior therapy for neglecting cognitive variables, and originally responding to it quite negatively. As I noted earlier in this book, I later reconsidered their stance, and was one of several Stony Brook faculty members that participated in an APA symposium, held in San Francisco in 1968, entitled "Cognitive processes in behavior modification."

The entry of cognition within behavior therapy circles seemed to pave the way for a still broader outlook. For example, in the 1970s, the clinical faculty at Stony Brook voted to expand the scope of the graduate therapy course, so that there would be some consideration of other therapeutic orientations. I was teaching that particular course at the time, and went back to many of the psychodynamic books that I had read as a graduate student. Much to my surprise, I began to note some interesting similarities, which began to spark my interest in rapprochement with other orientations.

Moreover, late-night discussions at the Association for the Advancement of Behavior Therapy (AABT) meetings with colleagues who were active contributors to the behavioral literature revealed that they had similarly been led to the conclusion that other orientations might help to make up for what behavior therapy lacked. Although they had not yet written about these private concerns, there nonetheless seemed to exist a well-respected "underground" (Wachtel, 1977).

During the first AABT meeting to be held in San Francisco in 1975, I decided that I would take the opportunity to broaden my horizons after the meetings, and I spent a week south of San Francisco in Esalan, the birthplace of gestalt therapy. I had at the time a two-sided suitcase, and packed half of it for AABT, and the other half for Esalan. Much less needed to be packed for Esalan.

This was all happening around the time that Davison and I were working on the manuscript for *Clinical Behavior Therapy* (Goldfried & Davison, 1976), and Davison was going through a similar professional self-exploration. In the introductory chapter to our book, we attempted to convey the need for greater professional openness when we suggested:

> in the attempt to expand knowledge and to improve the quality of our clinical services, it is time for behavior therapists to stop regarding themselves as an outgroup and instead to enter into serious and hopefully mutually fruitful dialogues with their nonbehavioral colleagues. Just as we firmly believe that there is much that behavior therapy can say to clinicians of other orientations, we reject the assumption that the slate should be wiped clean and that therapeutic innovation should be—and even can be—completely novel. (Goldfried & Davison, 1976, p. 15)

We went on to add:

> We firmly believe, however, that behavior therapy, when viewed as an experimental clinical approach to human difficulties, provides us with the most workable framework within which to expand the effectiveness of the behavior change process. (p. 17)

This began a desensitization process for me. Having now said it in print, my apprehension about voicing some of my concerns were reduced somewhat. Another major step in this process of disinhibition took place when I was demonstrating behavior therapy behind a one-way screen for graduate students. I was seeing a client on a weekly basis, where the primary focus was on the facilitation of assertiveness.

At various points during the therapy, I had to catch myself and stifle the temptation to say and do something that might not be considered "behavioral," but which I routinely made use of in my own clinical practice. After all, I was supposed to be demonstrating behavior therapy. One day, after discussing what had gone on during the session with the class, I confessed to them that I had been struggling with a dilemma, and proceeded to tell them what had been going on. They were most supportive, and encouraged me to do what I would usually do. This represented another significant incident in my "coming out."

Still another important step in my own personal/professional hierarchy occurred in the late 1970s, while I was spending a sabbatical leave in San Francisco. (There seems to be something about San Francisco that provides me with a supportive context for change.) During that year, I decided to prepare an article to submit to the *American Psychologist*, which would argue that the time was ripe for rapprochement across the orientations. The manuscript was accepted, and the article appeared shortly thereafter (Goldfried, 1980a).

BEHAVIOR THERAPISTS' REACTIONS TO INTEGRATION

The reaction of other behavior therapists to my involvement in rapprochement—and what has eventually developed into an integration movement—has been both positive and negative. Many welcomed having certain issues brought out into the open that had been confined to after-hour discussions over drinks at AABT meetings. Other behavior therapists reacted to the thought of introducing nonbehavioral concepts and methods into behavior therapy quite negatively.

Wilson (1982) once depicted behavior therapy as having moved from a focus on behavior in the 1950s and 1960s, to the incorporation of cognitive variables in the 1970s, suggesting that the 1980s would be the decade of affect. Little did I realize at the time that much of that affect would be directed at me.

In an issue of *the Behavior Therapist*, Adele Hayes and I (1989a) wrote about the possible contributions that other orientations might make to the practice of clinical behavior therapy. Although clearly acknowledging that behavioral interventions demonstrated greater effectiveness in the treatment of certain disorders (e.g., phobias and other anxiety disorders, childhood aggression, psychotic behaviors), we indicated that there still remained an array of clinical problems for which behavior therapy has not shown to be superior to other forms of treatment. One irate reader responded with an open letter, suggesting that our article reflected "a disturbing moral apathy toward the welfare of the consumer . . . and a seemingly blasé acceptance of treatments which are neither ethically acceptable or clinically correct" (Giles, 1989, p. 174). It was difficult to know how to respond to this criticism, except perhaps to caution that "an emotionally-based, schema-driven approach to reading the literature can be dangerous"— to ourselves as well as our clients (Goldfried & Hayes, 1989b, p. 175).

Among clinicians who are involved in conducting marital therapy, it is well accepted that sources of conflict can often be traced to miscommunication between individuals. This is certainly the case when therapists of different orientations try to communicate with each other. For example, in Arkowitz and Messer's (1984) edited volume, in which therapists from different orientations dialogued with each other, there was a lively interchange between Cyril Franks (a behavior therapist) and Leon Salzman (a psychodynamic therapist). The breakdown in communication between these two respected therapists seemed to be based on a lack of understanding of what was really involved in the therapeutic approach that the other advocated. Thus, Salzman (1984), in criticizing Franks, suggested: "It is unfortunate that some critics of psychoanalysis tend to use outmoded or disputed concepts as targets for attack" (p. 346). Ironically, Franks (1984a) independently called Salzman to task for referring to behavior therapy of the 1950s and 1960s when Salzman suggested that it was not a particularly useful approach with problems having a strong cognitive component. Although it might seem reasonable to make a more active effort to inform therapists of other orientations about our current status, a behavioral colleague of mine once objected to this prospect, exclaiming: "Why should we? What did they ever do for us?" The 1980s has indeed been the decade of affect.

Wilson (1990) has more recently suggested that it is unwise to incorporate any methods into behavior therapy that have not achieved empirical confirmation. I have a tremendous respect for Wilson's intellect and dedication; I did when he first arrived at Stony Brook as a graduate student, and have continued to maintain this respect over the years. Much to his credit, he also expressed his interest in the potential efficacy of interpersonal therapy for the treatment of bulimia, based on some recent outcome data provided by Fairburn (1988). Clearly, empirical confirmation of our interventions — regardless of the orientation — is crucial. Still, I would maintain that we often know more than we read in the literature.

Moreover, to suggest that the burden of proof is on those who identify with the orientation that gave rise to a particular method strikes me as being a bit too adversarial. If there is reason to believe that a procedure can make a clinical impact, even though it has not yet been demonstrated empirically, then I would think that *any* interested professional would be eager to see empirical confirmation. The fact that the orientation of origin was not behavioral should not preclude behavior therapists, who often constitute the majority of psychotherapy researchers, from testing its clinical efficacy.

CLINICAL OBSERVATIONS: THE CONTEXT OF DISCOVERY

In writing about scientific development, philosophers of science have made the distinction between the context of "discovery" and the context of "verification." Neal Miller (Bergin & Strupp, 1972) has applied this important distinction to his own work. Miller has indicated that when he has attempted to discover whether a phenomenon exists or not, he has followed hunches, has been free-wheeling, and usually has dispensed with control groups. Indeed, he had confessed that he has wasted much time and energy by being prematurely concerned with such methodological refinements. The primary purpose of this initial phase, says Miller, has been to convince himself that something exists. Once he has done that to his satisfaction, he has then moved on to the context of verification, where his goal was to convince his colleagues. I would maintain that for those of us interested in the development of empirically demonstrated therapy procedures, clinical observations represent the context of discovery (cf., Lazarus & Davison, 1971).

I do not mean to imply that behavior therapy should not be interested in extrapolating from basic principles of psychology. Nonetheless, we need to remember that not all basic research findings are as yet in, as our non-clinical colleagues will be quick to acknowledge. Thus, we are likely to fall short if we rely totally on extrapolating from the lab to the clinic. Moreover, my feeling has always been that sometimes the clinically-astute and empirically-grounded therapist can see things in the clinical situation that may not have as yet appeared in the literature. There are even times when clinical observations may be *more accurate* than the research literature. As noted in an earlier chapter, the research findings in the 1960s regarding relaxation training turned out to be wrong. These findings were obtained in the context of systematic desensitization dismantling studies, in which relaxation training alone was not found to be clinically effective. The fact of the matter was that the research designs did not provide a good enough parametric sampling of the relaxation induction, in that it wasn't thorough enough, and, moreover, not presented as a coping skill. Fortunately, our clients did not read the literature, and eventually got us to recognize that relaxation training may indeed be a very helpful clinical intervention. Ultimately, the research findings caught up with what clinicians had been noticing more informally.

Bannister and Fransella (1971) have warned us of the constant danger of having our research reflecting increasingly more precise procedures to test trivial issues. As they most astutely observe, such research is "born out of the literature and, no doubt, will be buried in it" (Bannister & Fransella, 1971, p. 193).

If we acknowledge that clinical observations can provide researchers with an important context of discovery, then we also may be able to entertain the possibility that these clinical observations may come from orientations other than our own. For example, there are a number of behavior therapists that find the clinical use of the gestalt two-chair technique to be extremely valuable, helping them to access "hotter" cognitions. There is now even some research to suggest that the two-chair technique is more effective than problem-solving in resolving conflict and facilitating decision-making (Clarke & Greenberg, 1986). Although I am not overjoyed to read findings that point to some potential limitations of problem-solving—an intervention with which I have had some personal involvement (D'Zurilla & Goldfried, 1971)—I find it difficult to negate them, especially since they are consistent with what I have seen clinically.

RESEARCH ON PSYCHOTHERAPY INTEGRATION

Recognizing the need for programmatic research in the general area of psychotherapy integration, NIMH sponsored a two-day workshop on this topic in 1986, the results of which have subsequently appeared in the 1988 volume of *Journal of Consulting and Clinical Psychology* (Wolfe & Goldfried, 1988). Among the various recommendations made, it was suggested that preliminary work be conducted on "desegregation" prior to actual controlled investigations of integrated treatments. The idea here is to conduct comparative analyses of both the common and unique processes that may operate across different so-called "pure form" therapies. Such research would take the form of process research, where the focus is on the mechanisms of change within different schools of thought. Although there might exist some common themes cutting across different orientations, it is also possible that parametric differences may be nested under certain commonalities. Once uncovered, such therapeutic processes need to be related to outcome, so that a compilation is made of effective change mechanisms—whatever their school of origin might have been. The ultimate goal is to develop integrated forms of treatment from these findings on the processes of change.

Our own research group at Stony Brook has been actively involved in such desegregation research. We have started with the common clinical strategy of therapeutic feedback, wherein the goal is to help clients become more aware of what they are doing and not doing, thinking and not thinking, and feeling and not feeling in various situations. Another way to think of such feedback is that the therapist is in the process of helping clients to "redeploy their attention" to clinically relevant aspects of their own functioning, and that of others with whom they interact.

Although we have started with the premise that different theoretical orientations share the strategy of providing feedback as a common strategy, we also believe that there are likely to be parametric variations associated with different schools of thought. Thus, while it is conceivable that both psychodynamic and cognitive-behavioral orientations are comparable in providing clients with feedback on the impact that they make on others, variations between these two schools of thought may exist with regard to who that other person is (i.e., the therapist vs. some other significant individual) or the time frame for providing such feedback (i.e., as it occurs within the session itself or between sessions).

In order to conduct such a comparative analysis, Cory Newman, Adele Hayes, and I (Goldfried, Newman & Hayes, 1989) have developed a coding system of therapeutic feedback. The system consists of guidelines for rating what the therapist may be focusing on during the course of a session, such as the client's thoughts, feelings, or actions, any possible links that may be made between these, connections that may be made between the client's functioning and the functioning of others, the people involved in the therapeutic focus, as well as the time frame.

In the process of developing this coding system, we obtained some preliminary findings on various data sets. The first study (Goldsamt, Goldfried, Hayes, & Kerr, 1992) looked at the similarities and differences among Beck, Meichenbaum, and Strupp, who conducted a demonstration session with the same patient — the case of Richard (Shostrom, 1986). Interestingly enough, our coders were able to guess which session transcript was Beck's, but could not differentiate between Strupp and Meichenbaum. We found that all three therapists were comparable in their focus on the impact that others made on the client (e.g., how they interpret the actions of others). However, in contrast to Beck, both Meichenbaum and Strupp were more likely to also point out the interpersonal impact that the client made on others — that is, what Richard was doing to possibly create certain interpersonal problems in his life. Beck seemed to be attempting to create more of a cognitive shift, as opposed to both a behavioral and cognitive change, as was the case with both Strupp and Meichenbaum.

A second study (Kerr, Goldfried, Hayes, & Goldsamt, 1989) made use of a data set obtained from David Shapiro and his colleagues in Sheffield, England (Hardy & Shapiro, 1985), which compared cognitive-behavior therapy with psychodynamic-interpersonal therapy. We found that both therapies made comparable use of intrapersonal and interpersonal links (i.e. focusing on connections within different aspects of the clients functioning—such as the interplay between thoughts and feelings—as well as connections made between the functioning of the client and that of someone else). Moreover, within both orientations, the predominant focus tended to be more interpersonal than intrapersonal.

A third study (Castonguay, Goldfried, Hayes, Raue, Wiser, & Shapiro, 1990) used the same Sheffield data set, but this time looked for the association between process variables and outcome measures. Although the previous study failed to find any differences in interpersonal links between the two orientations, this therapeutic focus tended to have more of a positive impact when conducted within the psychodynamic-interpersonal condition. Moreover, positive improvement in social adjustment within this form of therapy, but not cognitive-behavior therapy, was related to a therapeutic focus on the client's "transferential" reactions, such as the expected or imagined reaction that they had of other individuals, links between their functioning and the functioning of others, a focus on the therapist, stepping back and observing themselves more objectively, and to a lesser extent, a focus on their parent.

Still another finding of note had to do with the therapists' attempt to differentiate between the client's misperception of events and the way things "really" were (i.e., "reality-testing"). Within cognitive-behavior therapy, a near-significant positive correlation of .37 was obtained with symptom reduction, whereas a near-significant negative correlation of -.51 was obtained within the psychodynamic condition. I might add that the Ns were very small in this preliminary study, making it difficult to obtain traditional statistical significance, despite the size of the correlations. When we conducted a content analysis to try to better understand the nature of this surprising interaction, we found that the reality testing offered by behavior therapists typically consisted of the message "Things are not as *bad* as you think." By contrast, the psychodynamic therapists were communicating: "Things are not as *good* as you think."

These findings should be considered very preliminary, and our plan is to conduct a more detailed evaluation based on a larger data set being collected by Shapiro and his associates. We are also in the process of obtaining samples of significant sessions from experienced and highly-qualified cognitive-behavioral and psychodynamic-interpersonal therapists, as carried out in a naturalistic clinical setting, and additionally are looking at the nature of the therapeutic alliance and the experiencing levels of clients in these two forms of therapy.

CLOSING COMMENTS

My goal in this chapter has not been to downplay the contributions of behavior therapy. Far from it. I believe that behavior therapy has provided us with a unique and invaluable framework that has allowed us to see what other professionals could not. But to think that our approach to therapy — or any other — has the monopoly on truth is not only shortsighted, but dangerous.

It is part of our training as behavior therapists that we be responsive to what is there — in other words, to change as a result of what we see clinically and what the research reveals. There are times, however, when we as therapists are as culpable in our selective inattention to potentially helpful contributions from other orientations as our clients are in their difficulty in seeing what might make their lives better. As we move through the 1990s, which has been labeled by some, the decade of the brain, we can ill afford to maintain an overly-insular or antagonistic attitude to other psychosocial orientations.

In short, I believe it is time that we as behavior therapists seriously consider the possibility that our areas of weakness may be complemented by another orientation's strength. Bridges that are built between behavior therapy and other orientations, by definition, allow for movement both ways. Just as I have benefited in my own clinical and research activities from my ongoing dialogue with nonbehavioral colleagues (e.g., Goldfried & Wachtel, 1987), I have seen where they have changed as well.

My involvement in psychotherapy integration has been guided by two ongoing questions: (1) Are our interventions clinically relevant; that is, can I see it working in my own contacts with clients? (2) Has it been confirmed empirically; that is, does it work with other therapists under controlled experimental conditions? It is important to acknowledge, however, that the process of obtaining answers to this second question is often slow.

As indicated in the program for the 1990 AABT conference, behavior therapy is a "school of thought [that] is constantly evolving, resulting in a continuing need for the evaluation and consolidation of new information at all levels." In light of this, it would seem that behavior therapists are uniquely well-suited to entertain the possibility that procedures from other orientations might enhance our therapeutic effectiveness.

9

In Vivo Intervention or Transference?

Based on his observation that psychotherapists rarely discuss their clinical dilemmas in print, the British psychologist Windy Dryden (1985) conducted interviews with a number of therapists to examine those issues of uncertainty that typically arose during the course of their work. The interview that follows deals with my personal struggle to maintain an allegiance to a cognitive-behavioral orientation when it appears to conflict with what is called for by the case at hand:

WD: OK, Marvin, would you like to put your dilemma into your own words.

MG: The dilemma emerged within the context of a specific case and has re-emerged since that time with other clients that I've seen. As a result I can now frame the dilemma in broader terms. Let me start with the general case and then present the dilemma as it originally occurred, how it developed and how it influenced my thinking.

I have been approaching therapy from a cognitive-behavioral point of view, where, for the most part, the focus has been on the person's current life situation, rather than on his or her historical past. This leads to a review of the person's current life interactions and an emphasis on setting and evaluating homework assignments between sessions. The primary focus, then, is what goes on *between* the typical one-hour therapy session per week. At times, however, an indication of the person's problem may emerge *within* the therapeutic interaction. The dilemma here is being able to recognize when

135

this occurs and being able to decide when to focus on this in-session phenomenon rather than on what goes on between sessions.

WD: So it's a question of when to shift one's perspective from looking for maintaining factors of a person's problems that exist within the person's current life, i.e. a between-sessions focus, to considering that certain maintaining factors might be right there in the room with you, i.e. a within-session focus.

MG: That's right. One of the constraints against making this shift, which perhaps we can discuss later, is that once we focus on what is going on within the session and within the therapist-client interaction, we are then making use of therapeutic orientation that is not typically part of the realm of cognitive-behavior therapy, but is much more psychodynamic in orientation. This may very well account for the fact that many cognitive-behavior therapists are limited in their ability to recognize this phenomenon when it occurs within the therapy session.

WD: I wonder whether this in fact has to be the case. Just because cognitive-behavioral therapists choose to pay attention to material that is going on between therapist and patient, does their conceptualization necessarily have to be psychodynamic?

MG: No it doesn't. But I must confess to experiencing a certain amount of initial self-consciousness when I shifted the focus to what was going on within the session itself, even though conceptually I can reconcile this with my more cognitive-behavioral orientation. Maybe this reconciliation might become clear after I have given a specific clinical example of it.

The first time this occurred—and I have become sensitized to it since then because I recognize that it occurs rather frequently—was with a 51-year-old male accountant with whom I was working. This man had a problem of depression, not only in his current life situation, but had a long history of intermittent depression since being a teenager. In his current life situation he felt trapped, both in his relationship with his boss at work and in his relationship with his wife. He felt he was being controlled by others and was powerless to lead his own life. He had a great need to please others. The result of all this was a chronic sense of depression. Since he felt unable to *directly* control many aspects of his life situation, he would act in a passive–aggressive manner by "fooling around" with other women or by not doing his job properly. This led to additional problems in his life, such as feeling guilty about his job performance and his extramarital affairs.

My dilemma started to emerge when I presented him with a cognitive-behavioral conceptualization of his problems and a formulation of the treatment plan—both of which he initially accepted. He had been, I should add, in analytically-oriented therapy for several years prior to this, but wanted a more structured and directive therapy, which was why he sought me out. Yet, once we identified the problem of unassertiveness as being at the core of many of his problems, and once I suggested that this was an area he needed to work on, therapy never got off the ground, despite his initial agreement. There was always something that would interfere. He would be forever bringing up other problems that would divert the course of the therapeutic focus. This was partly due to the fact that there were a lot of issues going on in his life. It was also partly due to his obsessional style, in that it was hard for him to let go of things. His very deliberate and slow style meant that the sessions were sometimes very painful to get through. And part of it might have been a function of the fact that he was socialized to act as a patient in analytic therapy.

When I first tried to get some notion as to what the dilemma was, it was that he wanted help and wanted structure, but at the same time he didn't want these things. He would ask me questions such as "What shall I do?" or "How can I handle situations differently?" and then when I would give a suggestion within a didactic, supervisory role, he would not always follow through on this. So there would be periods where he would start to assert himself more with people in his life, would back off, and other problems would crop up. He would then need to talk more about trying to understand why he was having some reactions, wanting to gain greater insight into his feelings. He thus wanted a more intrapsychic focus, rather than one that was more overt, behavioral and performance based. In thinking further about this kind of double bind that I was being placed in, i.e., with him asking for help from me, yet not really wanting it, it eventually became clear that the reason he didn't want help or suggestions from me, even though he asked for it, was that to him, accepting help meant that he could not help himself. Furthermore, he wanted to deal more with a lot of his past experience and with a lot of the subtleties of his emotional reactions. As I was trying to be more structured in helping him with corrective experiences that might advance his assertiveness and make him feel better, there was a kind of tension between us as to what the direction of therapy should be. It ultimately emerged that he was furious at me for controlling the therapy and not giving him what he wanted. His anger would take the form of his coming in and telling me of all the terrible things he experienced during the course of the week, rather than reporting any success experiences he had. When I tried to put the focus on his successes, he would initially comply; only later on did he realize that he was very, very, angry with me.

WD: So it sounds as if you were getting a double message from him.

MG: Yes. It took me a while before I realized what was underneath this double message. Even before I gained an understanding of what it was, I started to resolve this particular dilemma by becoming more passive within the session. I just let him take it wherever he wanted to.

WD: You were stepping out of role.

MG: Yes, I was stepping out of the role of cognitive-behavior therapist who was teaching somebody coping skills. In the process of stepping out of role and really letting him take the lead, it became more apparent to both of us that he was reacting against me. He was acting in a similar passive-aggressive manner with me as he had with other people in life. For example he contacted an old girlfriend, after telling me that he was going to stop his extramarital affairs. He went back on his antidepressant medication, after we both agreed that he no longer needed it. These were some of the indirect ways in which he expressed his anger towards me. After a while, the focus of the therapy shifted to what was going on between us.

WD: I wonder to what extent the difficulty you experienced in stepping out of the role of a cognitive-behavior therapist who was there to teach coping skills was accentuated by the fact that you have written on this topic and made a public statement on that score. Namely that the core of successful therapy is the degree to which the therapist can teach the client coping skills. Was this a factor at all?

MG: Well, I don't think so, because I would still ascribe to that notion. And I still believe that the teaching of coping skills is what good therapy is all about. The problem here is how to define "teaching." Perhaps a better way to conceptualize this point is that the core of therapy is that the client *learn* coping skills. If we look at it that way then, as therapists, we became free to explore different methods of facilitating the client's learning.

WD: It still sounds as if you experienced some discomfort about stepping out of a more active and structured kind of role. Could you articulate this more?

MG: I think what happened was that I became less active and more passive. It was important for me to be more of an observer of what was going on in the interaction, and less of a participant. As I became more of an observer, I was better able to see that what was going on in the interaction was very much the same kind of thing that was going on outside in his relationship with his boss and his wife when they told him to do things. He resented that, did not want to comply, but felt powerless. And because he felt that there was nothing he could do, he would become depressed, but also act out in passive–aggressive ways. As I became less directive, it became quite apparent to me that this was going on. Because I was a participant — too much of a participant, and not enough of an observer — I hadn't been aware that this was the issue.

WD: I am still not sure what the basis of the difficulty or the discomfort was in moving from a participant role to an observer role.

MG: Well, part of the difficulty was that it was harder for me to be an observer. It is much easier to see things outside of ourselves than it is to see ourselves in the context of an interaction. I think that part is self-evident, in much the same way that clients find it difficult to see their own contribution to some of their life dilemmas, and require an external observer in the form of a therapist to help provide them with that perspective. So I think that is the nature of the beast; indeed it is "biological" in origin. Because our eyeballs are situated in our head, it is easier to see things outside of ourselves; were they retractable so that we could look back on ourselves, we could give ourselves a clearer perspective on ourselves.

WD: Yes. I accept that. Although if you were a psychodynamically trained therapist, that is precisely what you would be trained to observe.

MG: Yes. And that, no doubt, was a factor that made me feel uneasy about doing that. I am certainly well aware of the fact that this is the essence of a psychodynamic approach to therapy, and it was almost as if I was now abrogating my cognitive-behavioral allegiance and taking up a therapeutic stance that has been used by an alternative camp. I had been aware that this is an ongoing dilemma that I had experienced for a number of years in doing therapy. This may be getting off the track a bit, but let me just add a brief tangent here. Over the years when I conducted demonstrations of therapy behind a one-way screen for students taking courses in behavior therapy, I noticed that I was very constrained in what I said and did. What I said and did while I was doing a demonstration was very different from what I would do if I wasn't conducting a demonstration. So it became apparent to me that I had been deviating from the constraints of a certain orientation over the years, and these experiences would bring home this awareness to me.

WD: You became aware of the discrepancy of your public image from what you privately did in therapy.

MG: Exactly. As I say, this had been going on for a number of years, and is in fact one of the things that got me interested in cognitive-behavior therapy. It was apparent that cognitive factors played an important role in therapy, and that the more classic 1960s behavior therapy was not adequate to deal with what went on clinically. So, my whole professional career as a behavior therapist has been characterized by many dilemmas all along the way.

WD: Coming back to the case. Did that shift in emphasis help resolve the block that seemed to have emerged?

MG: Yes. As I said, what happened was that the client's resentment towards my structuring the sessions in ways that went counter to what he wanted started to come to the fore. A lot of the feelings that he had vis-à-vis other people were now expressed directly and openly to me; namely, that he felt powerless to control the session and direct its course, fearful of what I might do if he stated his opinion. He was enraged, but felt unable to express that anger. As we focused on this over a period of several sessions, he ultimately did tell me how angry he was. This was a very powerful and dramatic experience for him, because nothing terrible happened. We got through that and re-established a therapeutic alliance with the two of us working jointly on his problems. This situation, rather than the one where it was him against me — where I was overpowering him as it were — together with the fact that he could express his anger and learn that nothing had happened, opened up a whole dimension for him.

WD: It sounds as if he was able to test out a pretty fundamental assumption with you that if he were to express his feeling then terrible things might happen, and yet he actually learned to the contrary.

Going on from that, cognitive-behavior therapists have not, in the main, addressed themselves very much to the notion of exploring the therapist–client interaction. I wonder to what extent you were operating under that notion with this man that what cognitive-behavior therapists are supposed to do is to work on relationships between the client and the client's significant others rather than between the client and themselves.

MG: My sense is that this is the typical procedure. At least I have not seen too much written about cognitive-behavior therapy making use of the interaction. Now in books like *Clinical Behavior Therapy*, which Gerald Davison and I originally published in the mid 1970s, we recognized the importance of the therapist–client interaction as a potential sample of the client's relationships. *When* to deal with this relationship presents a different question. I had always operated on the assumption that when clients bring in problems they experienced between sessions, we would work on that. Since that is closest to the criterion that we are working towards, that would seem better. In the case I've outlined, our relationship was interfering, so it had to be dealt with. Once we did deal with it, in fact, the client started to become much more assertive with other people and very willingly engaged in assertion training, focusing on people in his life situation apart from myself. Not only did we dispense with the issue of who controlled the course of therapy, but the experience of having risked stating his preferences to me in very forceful terms (he was aggressive and not assertive) and realizing that nothing terrible happened provided him with what Alexander and French (1946) described as a "corrective emotional experience." He felt less depressed after having regained control over the direction of his therapy and he began to see the connection in a much more personal way between assertiveness and the absence of depression. Initially, when he accepted this formulation, he did so only superficially; he was still operating on the notion that he needed to gain insight prior to any change in behavior. But here, he saw something from his own personal experience that convinced him that he could become less depressed in a particular situation when he had his say.

WD: You mentioned earlier that this experience with this particular client sensitized you to the whole issue of the importance of dealing with the therapist–client relationship when appropriate. You mention this particular case in the sense that the interactional dynamics between you and the client interfered with treatment. Are you saying then that when there is, if you like, an obvious resistance, then that is the time for cognitive-behavior therapists to address themselves to the therapist–client relationship? Or are you going further than that and saying that as a matter of course, cognitive-behavior therapists would be wise to consider the here-and-now relationship as a microcosm in which the client's problems might occur?

MG: I think the latter. The thing that sensitized me in this particular case was the fact that therapy was not proceeding. I think that there are other times when it would be wise to deal with the interaction between the therapist and client as a potential sample — a microcosm of the client's problem. I think it stands to reason that, under certain circumstances, and with certain individuals, the therapist will serve as a stimulus for the client's problems in much the same way as others in the person's life will serve as stimuli. To assume that there is no stimulus value for the therapist or the therapy interaction is to assume that therapy operates in a vacuum in a person's life, when in fact it is a very salient event. Consequently, I think that we should look at it much more seriously at times even when it does not seem to be interfering with the progress of therapy. If "dealing with the transference" is an aversive conceptualization, perhaps we can think of it as "in vivo work." We know that in vivo interventions are much more powerful than imaginal or described ones. So if we can look at the person's actions right at the time — when they are being upset about something, or when they are being inhibited and cannot act in a given way or say something within the session itself — we have broadened our therapeutic focus. This, incidentally, is not at all inconsistent with a cognitive-behavioral orientation, even though another orientation might have "gotten there first."

WD: Right, psychodynamic therapists got there first, in talking about the importance of exploring such "here-and-now" data but the inferences they made about such data would be foreign to cognitive-behavioral therapists.

MG: When you look at the notion of transference from a Sullivanian point of view, it is much closer to a cognitive-behavioral perspective. He spoke in terms of "parataxic distortions," namely that individuals have certain misconceptions of significant people that they developed early in life and carry with them to other significant people later in life. I don't think that this is a very high-level inference that involves "repetition compulsion" or "unresolved needs" or any other kinds of constructs of a drive-related, motivational nature. It is really just descriptive.

WD: Exactly. If I can move the tangent slightly, you are involved at the moment in developing the Society for the Exploration of Psychotherapy Integration — SEPI. The way you have just spoken seems to me as if you are saying: "Well look, I am still a cognitive-behavioral therapist, but I have expanded the range of data to which I am going to attend." Would you say that was accurate?

MG: Yes.

WD: I wonder what range of experiences may actually lead you to change your self-description as a cognitive-behavioral therapist to, for want of a better word, an integrationist. I want to bring out the tensions that exist between adhering to a particular perspective as opposed to moving into the new area of psychotherapy integrationism.

MG: That is an interesting question, and indeed another dilemma that I am often faced with when I work with clients. I ask myself, and also them, what range of experiences does one have to go through to change one's view of oneself? I think that it is a hard question for anyone to answer. It's hard for me to answer that about myself. I know that the existence of SEPI makes it easier for me to openly acknowledge that I am struggling with some of these dilemmas, mainly because I am in very good company. Having a reference group of other people whom I respect and who are similarly concerned with these issues makes it easier for me to openly acknowledge that I'm grappling with these issues as well.

There is another problem, though, in that there exists no other orientation with which I can identify. I have my own set of idiosyncratic notions, but it is really far from complete, and I would not dignify it by giving it a name or even by describing it in writing. It is still in its very early stages of formulation. It is so incomplete that I really can't identify myself as "being that."

WD: Personally do you hope that the formation of SEPI, with its attempt to bring together "fellow strugglers," will be a step towards the situation where people do not label themselves as belonging to particular schools of therapy?

MG: I would hope so.

WD: So we might actually see Marvin Goldfried at some point in the future stop describing himself as a cognitive-behavior therapist, because you would share that aim?

MG: Yes. I honestly cannot say that I am terribly optimistic that this might happen in my professional lifetime.

WD: I would like to think that this interview might perhaps hasten things on a little.

MG: Well, maybe, but by its very definition, the integrative approach involves an integration of varying schools of thought in some sophisticated way—rather than the situation where a therapist says: "I'll use a technique from orientation A and a technique from orientation B, etc." We need to have a more integrative model of human functioning and human change, and I don't think any comprehensive one yet exists.

WD: So you doubt whether integration will occur at a theoretical level?

MG: Yes. I think for integration to occur, there needs to be a totally new theoretical structure about how people change that can account for the varying procedures that seem to work. The original behavioral model was inadequate, as is the contemporary cognitive-behavioral one. For example, it does not adequately deal with the emotions. An increasing number of cognitive-behavioral therapists are recognizing this, and a few of them are getting interested in the work done by experiential therapists. I find this development interesting and intriguing. I've had some fascinating experiences at an experiential-behavioral workshop sponsored by the National Institute of Mental Health. It was organized by Barry Wolfe to bring together a group of behavior therapists and a group of experiential therapists to dialogue on the processes of change and how such processes can be adequately investigated. As a result of this workshop, it became apparent to me that the affective components of a client's functioning are not adequately dealt with by cognitive-behavioral methods.

WD: So you are hopeful that a series of these dialogues will actually bring together people from different schools so that the identification of a superordinate theory may actually emerge, that may actually help people to become integrationists?

MG: Yes. I think, though, that it would be misleading to expect that a superordinate theory can be a combination of existing theories. I think that many people are put off by the interest in therapeutic integration because they believe that it is taking psychoanalytic therapy, behavior therapy and experiential orientations, and putting them into a blender and coming up with something that integrates it all. That is clearly not what it is all about. What we need is to reach some consensus about the common principles that operate across the therapies. Once we have identified a set of these principles that seem to be comprehensive, then perhaps inductively we can come up with some higher level theoretical explanation that takes them into account. It is this middle level that we need to work at initially rather than at the highly abstract theoretical level or at the lower level of technique.

For example, if we look at the notion of helping clients achieve awareness, and look at subcategories under the general rubric of awareness, we can probably come up with principles that therapists could agree on as operating in the change process. If we take the instance where therapists help clients become aware that some of the unpleasant things in their lives—such as negative reactions from others—occur as the result of some behavior pattern on their part, then I would speculate that most clinicians, regardless of orientation, would say that this is an important therapeutic task. Once we can come up with many of these kinds of principles, especially ones that have support from basic findings in psychology, I think that the enterprise of therapy is really going to advance beyond the point where it is now.

10

Can Contributions from Other Orientations Complement Behavior Therapy?

The field of psychotherapy in the 1980s was highlighted by a rapidly developing movement toward integration and eclecticism. Faced with the pragmatics of clinical work, an increasing number of therapists have expressed dissatisfaction with the use of a single orientation, acknowledging that no one approach can explain or generate interventions for the broad range of clinical phenomena they observe in practice. As a result, clinicians from a variety of orientations are borrowing techniques from other schools of therapy in an effort to enhance their clinical effectiveness.

THE CLINICAL NEED

Garfield and Kurtz's (1976) well-known survey of clinical psychologists indicated that even at that time more psychotherapists in the United States designated themselves as eclectic than as belonging to any given psychotherapy school. When queried, the most frequent reason they gave for using more than one framework was based on the demands of clinical work (Garfield & Kurtz, 1977). More recent surveys have documented that between one-third to one-half of practicing clinicians classify themselves as eclectic (see Norcross, 1986a; Mahoney, Norcross, Prochaska, & Missar, 1987).

147

Surveys of behavior therapists reveal that they too have expressed dissatisfaction with practicing exclusively within the confines of their orientation. For example, in a questionnaire submitted to leading cognitive and noncognitive behavior therapists, Mahoney (1979) found that, overall, these clinicians were not satisfied with the adequacy of their current understanding of human behavior. In fact, on a 7-point scale (1 equals not at all satisfied, 7 equals very satisfied), the average rating of satisfaction was less than 2. Moreover, cognitive and noncognitive behavior therapists did not differ significantly in their ratings of satisfaction. This dissatisfaction among behavior therapists may have increased their willingness to integrate interventions from nonbehavioral orientations in an effort to better serve their clients.

In addition to the dissatisfaction expressed by practicing clinicians, most major reviews of the treatment outcome literature have returned the verdict that no brand of therapy has been demonstrated to be significantly and consistently more effective than its competitors (see reviews by Bergin & Lambert, 1978; Luborsky, Singer, & Luborsky, 1975; Smith, Glass, & Miller, 1980). In a critical review of the outcome literature, Lambert, Shapiro, and Bergin (1986) concluded that although behavior therapy, cognitive therapy, and eclectic combinations of these have been demonstrated to have superior outcomes to traditional verbal therapies with phobias, compulsions, and other difficult problems (e.g., childhood aggression, psychotic behaviors, stuttering), this superior outcome is by no means the general case. Thus, they hold that the movement of clinicians toward eclecticism is a healthy response to the empirical evidence.

Proposed Solutions

In the absence of a unified and empirically based model of psychotherapy, clinicians seem to be practicing the "technical eclecticism" espoused by Lazarus some years ago. Lazarus (1967, 1977) maintained that clinicians can use techniques from various therapy orientations without necessarily subscribing to the theoretical underpinnings associated with these methods. The selection of techniques, he argued, should be based on empirical, not theoretical grounds. In short, therapists should be guided by what works rather than by the consistency of the techniques with their theoretical orientation.

Where prescriptive treatments have been delineated, the responsible clinician certainly should employ those interventions demonstrated to be effective for the case at hand. For instance, given the consensus on the efficacy of behavior therapy for anxiety disorders articulated at the NIMH-SUNY research conference (Barlow & Wolfe, 1981), a clinician who does not employ a behavioral treatment for an obsessive-compulsive client is clearly negligent. However, Goldfried and Safran (1986) caution that psychotherapists who are guided exclusively by what works are mere technicians. By contrast, clinicians who understand why interventions work are able to select methods based on an understanding of the psychotherapy process and the principles of therapeutic change. The knowledge of both orientation-specific and more transtheoretical change processes is necessary to guide therapists who choose not to operate from within the confines of a single theoretical orientation in the selection of interventions.

Goldfried and Safran (1986) contend that the task of developing an integrated perspective on psychotherapy must take place from both the "top down" and from the "bottom up." Although scholarly examinations of the similarities and differences among different psychotherapy traditions can be conducted at a conceptual level, it is essential that empirical comparisons be made at the level of clinical practice. In addition, these two types of knowledge must be linked in a systematic way. Moreover, they hold that the advancement of the field of psychotherapy depends on contributions from clinicians and researchers alike. The invaluable experience of the practicing clinician cannot be overlooked, but it must also be linked to empirical research so that this source of information can add to a reliable, empirically based body of knowledge. Similarly, the growing methodological sophistication of the researcher is of little use if not linked to significant and ecologically valid clinical phenomena. In short, our knowledge about what works in therapy must be rooted in clinical observations, but must also have an empirical base. Clinical observations from a variety of therapy orientations need to be clearly articulated and examined empirically, so as to increase our understanding of the therapy change process. Operating at this level of abstraction, the clinician can select interventions on the basis of their potential for implementing a given principle of therapeutic change, rather than on the random use of whatever is found to work.

Addressing himself to behavior therapists in particular, Levis

(1988) lamented that because clinical observations and wisdom have been disregarded by many behavior therapists, they remain ignorant of potentially useful treatment-related findings reported in the nonbehavioral literature. Psychoanalytic theory, Levis goes on to argue, remains a dominant influence in the study of psychopathology because it addresses itself to a number of commonly observed clinical phenomena that the behavioral movement has denied or considered unimportant. Hence, psychodynamic concepts—however ambiguous or limited they may be—may provide some useful leads for behavior therapists attempting to broaden their clinical scope. Despite the "conditioned emotional reaction" that many of us have developed against anything that appears to be Freudian in origin, Levis argues that many psychodynamic concepts are consistent with the tenets of behaviorism. He exhorts that if behavior therapy is to make a long-lasting contribution, it must provide conceptual models of psychopathology that not only advance the field by linking clinical observations to research, but also explain the repeatedly observed clinical realities.

The present chapter is in response to cognitive-behavior therapists' attempts to increase their clinical effectiveness and to broaden the scope of problems with which they can intervene. Toward this goal, we examine the clinical utility of several concepts and techniques that have emerged from other orientations and, where possible, link them to available research findings.

A Look at Some Useful Nonbehavioral Concepts

When theorists and researchers from different therapy orientations discuss the nature of therapeutic change and how it can be brought about, it becomes apparent that many aspects of the nonbehavioral therapies are not nearly as inconsistent with those of behavior therapy as one might think. Strupp (1988), a noted clinician, theorist, and researcher from the psychodynamic tradition, describes several psychodynamic concepts in a provocative paper entitled "What is Therapeutic Change?" His views on the role of the therapeutic relationship, cognitive shifts in the patient's perspective, and the role of affect in the change process will be discussed as they relate to a behavioral perspective on these issues, and considered in light of relevant research findings. This comparison is intended to highlight the consistency of certain aspects of the psychodynamic conceptualization of the therapeutic change process with those of the behavioral tradition. In addition, a discussion of the role of affect in therapeutic change will be used to examine the utility of integrating concepts from the more experiential therapies with behavior therapy. Through a consideration of the extent to which these nonbehavioral concepts are compatible with a cognitive-behavioral perspective, we may gain concepts that bring with them the particular strengths of a different perspective and hopefully, the potential of increasing our clinical efficacy.

The therapeutic relationship. The importance of the psychoanalytic notion of "transference" in the therapeutic change process has received an increasing amount of attention in the psychotherapy literature. Strupp (1988) asserts that one of the most powerful tools at the therapist's disposal is the ability to utilize his or her own emotional reactions that are engendered in transactions with the client and to present this feedback in the context of the current interaction. These transference issues, he continues, provide some of the most readily observed data that can ever become available to the client and to the therapist. Moreover, Strupp continues, interpretations in this context have the potential of effecting meaningful and lasting changes.

As suggested elsewhere, Goldfried (1985, 1988a) contends that it is reasonable to assume that the therapist will, at times, serve as a "stimulus" for the client's problems. Moreover, "to assume that there is no stimulus value for the therapist or for the therapy interaction is to assume that therapy operates in a vacuum within the client's life, when in fact, it is often the most salient" (Goldfried, 1985, p. 71). Yet, some behavior therapists may be reluctant to focus on the client-therapist relationship because it means that they will be dealing with the X-rated concept of "transference" (the dreaded "T-word"). As noted in Chapter 9, it is as carrying out an *in vivo* intervention, which, as we know, is more powerful than described or imaginal interventions. To the extent that the client's problem is of an interpersonal nature that shows itself in his or her relationship with the therapist, it seems foolhearty for us to ignore what is going on within the therapeutic relationship simply because it comes close to an intervention that is typically associated with a psychodynamic orientation.

Furthermore, the psychoanalytic lore about the transference phenomenon has been linked to important new developments in the social cognition literature (see Singer, 1988; Westen, 1988). In a compelling examination of transference from an information-processing perspective, Westen (1988) attempts to integrate social cognition and psychodynamic concepts to demonstrate the therapeutic importance of transference. Specifically, transference is described as a mechanism for the assessment and alteration of dysfunctional scripts, expectancies, and wishes, and for the uncovering of state-dependent memories and schema-triggered affects.

Westen construes one aspect of transference as the activation of scripts. Scripts are schemas embodying knowledge of stereotyped event sequences that are used to comprehend social events and organize action (Abelson, 1981; Schank & Abelson, 1977). Scripts become routinized, and do not necessarily require conscious attention. They are activated when events or cues in the social environment match certain features encoded in a given script. Given that the therapist or the therapeutic relationship may activate a particular script, the transference may be an invaluable source of information about the client's interpersonal action patterns, as well as their assumptions/expectancies/wishes about the world. The therapist can use the transference to look beyond the client's self-report and use an in vivo sample as a powerful demonstration of how the client interacts with significant others, and what that individual, in reality, expects and desires from them. By making these scripts, expectancies, and wishes explicit and conscious, the therapist can help the individual to examine and change them if they are erroneous or maladaptive.

Another use of transference, suggests Westen, is the uncovering of state-dependent memories and schema-triggered affect. The client's expression of positive or negative feelings toward the therapist may reflect the activation of a given schema or script and its associated affect. The perceived similarity between aspects of the therapist or therapy situation and the characteristics of a cognitive prototype activates the schema associated with the prototype, as well as the affect associated with it. Fiske (1982) demonstrated that the greater the number of prototypic features that characterize the stimulus person, the more likely the schema-based affect is to be triggered and the more intensely it will be experienced. Thus, an important aspect of therapy may be to trace the affect expressed toward the therapist to its origins, in order to examine whether the affect attached to a given category is an appropriate one, or one that needs to be reworked.

The use of transference as outlined by Strupp (1988), Goldfried

(1985, 1988a) and Westen (1988) enlists the active participation of the client and utilizes an in vivo sample of their social interactions. Given the findings on the effectiveness of in vivo interventions. it seems that behavior therapists would agree that activating feelings, interactional patterns, and schemas in session would have a greater impact than simply talking about those that occur outside of the sessions with others.

Cognitive shifts. Strupp (1988) construes psychotherapy as a learning process that occurs primarily in the context of the therapeutic relationship rather than through the provision of extratherapy experiences, the hallmark of the more behavioral approaches. According to this view, the therapist provides new experiences in a benign interpersonal context, thus enabling the client to modify previous learning and acquire different patterns of thinking, feeling, and behaving. Consistent with Beck's (1985) view of cognitive processing as a common pathway through which various systems of psychotherapy produce therapeutic results, Strupp holds that therapy is a corrective experience that involves a shift in the client's perspective and cognitive reorganization of some sort.

Strupp's discussion of the need to change one's "assumptive world" leads him to acknowledge the contributions of Beck and Ellis, although he asserts that working with current faulty belief systems alone is not sufficient. An emphasis on the historical origins of these beliefs, Strupp maintains, is also necessary if one is to understand the effects that they continue to exert on current functioning. Interestingly, Beck and Emery (1985) have stated that at times the therapist needs to present the client with the distinction between certain beliefs that were appropriate in the past and those that are relevant to one's current life situation. Work has also been done in Beck's clinic examining the role of imagery in helping the client to retrieve and ultimately restructure schemas from childhood that may still be exerting an influence on current functioning (J. Beck, personal communication, January 22, 1988). Thus, although they represent two different theoretical orientations, Strupp and Beck seem to agree that by helping clients to become aware that they hold certain beliefs, that these beliefs are based on earlier experiences, and that these views may no longer be relevant to their current lives, the therapist may be encouraging them to shift their perspective and to take the steps needed to make certain changes.

The role of affect.   Strupp (1988) considers therapeutic change ultimately to be forged in the affective context. Change is thought to be brought about by "insight," which is the "affective experiencing and cognitive understanding of the current maladaptive patterns of behavior that repeat childhood patterns of interpersonal conflict" (Strupp & Binder, 1984, pp. 24–25). The client's "insights" become most potent when one's current experience, preferably in relation to the therapist, evokes the painful emotions that are thought to be associated with one's earlier faulty learning. For change to occur, Strupp asserts that the affect, the faulty belief, and the current interpersonal experience must come together in the here-and-now.

Cognitive-behavior therapists have similarly become more appreciative of the role of emotional factors in the change process. In his presidential address to AABT, Wilson (1982) reviewed the history of behavior therapy as moving from an emphasis on overt behavior in the 1950s and 1960s to the addition of cognition in the 1970s, and predicted a new emphasis on "affect in the eighties" (p. 298). Recognizing the increasing evidence for the importance of affect in the therapeutic change process, Beck and Weishaar (1989) maintain that the cognitive constellations that underlie a given problem can become accessible and are modifiable only with affective arousal. This shaft may be reflective of what seems to be a general tendency within the field to recognize the importance of emotional processes in human functioning, as well as the specific role they may play in creating therapeutic change (see Greenberg & Safran, 1987).

The increased emphasis on the role of affective arousal in the change process is consistent with recent findings in cognitive research. In a comprehensive review, Singer and Salovey (1988) concluded that there is a considerable body of research to support Bower's (1981) elegant network theory of affect, which deals with state-dependent memory. Bower's theory suggests that the retrieval of material is enhanced by reinstating the mood that the individual experienced when the material was originally encoded. Additionally, the greater the intensity of the mood state, the greater the accessibility of the cognitive-affective network. An application of these data to the clinical realm suggests that affect-enhancing interventions may facilitate the recall of previously inaccessible cognitive and affective material, thus making these schemas more amenable to re-evaluation. Consistent with Strupp's (1988) views, it would seem that when therapeutic interventions are associated with emotional arousal, the likelihood of affective, cognitive, and related behavioral change may be the greatest.

In an article on "cold" and "hot" cognitions, Safran and Greenberg (1986) cite a variety of procedures that can be useful for increasing affective arousal and accessing associated cognitive material. These procedures range from role plays, to imagery techniques and *in vivo* procedures, to working with thoughts and feelings that emerge in the context of a therapeutic relationship.

An affect-enhancing intervention that may be particularly relevant to behavior therapy is the gestalt two-chair technique (Greenberg, 1984; Perls, 1973), which may be used to enhance the effectiveness of such cognitive-behavioral techniques as rational restructuring. Rational restructuring may be construed as facilitating an implicit, internal dialogue between the realistic and unrealistic sides of an individual. As suggested in Chapter 6, the two-chair exercise may be used to make this internal dialogue external, explicit, and more affectively charged.

In the use of the two-chair procedure, the task of the client is to carry out a dialogue between the rational and irrational sides of themselves, changing chairs each time they switch sides. Several clinicians (e.g., Goldfried, 1988b; Greenberg & Safran, 1987) who have used this procedure in their practice, have noted a greater amount of affective arousal with the two-chair technique than with mere discussion. The former elicits what might be considered "hotter" cognitions than the latter. Given the affective arousal associated with the two-chair technique, previously inaccessible affective and cognitive material may be accessed, thereby facilitating restructuring. Although the testimonies of the effectiveness of the two-chair technique are consistent with Bower's (1981) network theory of affect, the extent to which this technique enhances rational restructuring, as typically implemented, clearly needs to be examined empirically.

The two-chair technique has been demonstrated to be superior to problem-solving therapy (D'Zurilla & Goldfried, 1971) in facilitating conflict resolution and decision-making (Clarke & Greenberg, 1986). The basic premise of problem-solving therapy is that when a person experiences the negative affect and paralysis associated with indecision, these feelings should be set aside and the problem should be approached through a rational examination of the issue at hand. By contrast, the basic premise of the gestalt two-chair technique is that when faced with the negative experiences associated with indecision, the person must attend to the feelings being experienced in order to bring unacknowledged aspects of the experience (e.g., needs) into awareness. This awareness of the different aspects of the negative experience and the dialogue between them is believed to lead to an integration and conflict resolution. In an integrative spirit, Clarke and Greenberg (1986) suggest that the problem-solving approach may complement the affective approach by providing a way to generate strategies for taking action that can implement the decision, once it is made.

CONCLUSIONS

In a discussion of the nature and process of therapeutic change, a consistent principle that emerges across therapeutic orientations is that, whenever possible, it is important to work with events using in vivo, affectively charged material. Psychodynamic theory has suggested that the client's responses to the therapist or the therapeutic relationship may be used as a concrete, verifiable, and affect-laden sample of the person's interactions with significant others. Additionally, cognitive-behavior therapists are beginning to recognize that cognitive skills and restructuring may be enhanced by uncovering the historical origins of currently operating negative schemas and relating them to current functioning. Finally, given recent findings in the cognitive literature, behavior therapists are also beginning to recognize the important role of affect in the change process and thus may be more amenable to using such affect-enhancing interventions as the gestalt two-chair technique.

This chapter is intended to encourage behavior therapists to look to other therapy orientations in the hope of increasing their clinical effectiveness. In line with the integrationist approach, clinical observations and techniques from nonbehavioral orientations were examined from the perspective of how therapeutic change occurs. They were evaluated for their consistency with behavior therapy and with relevant empirical data.

An integrationist approach such as this serves to point clinicians to contributions that may have originated from outside of their theoretical orientation and to testable hypotheses that may have otherwise gone unnoticed. Behaviorally-oriented researchers, in particular, have the methods to subject these new hypotheses to empirical scrutiny, but they are unlikely to do so unless they attend to ideas developed outside of their orientation. As Kazdin (1986a) convincingly argues:

> A major advance in the field is the attempt among many to shed rival conceptual positions and the promulgation of narrow orientations or techniques. Many researchers wish to reach a consensus about strategies that apply broadly across techniques and orientations. The explicit movement toward integration reflects an ecumenical spirit among researchers and clinicians. Integrationistism holds special promise for the evaluation of psychotherapy. (p. 281)

Integrationism was born out of clinical need and a dissatisfaction with the fruits of a previously segregated professional community. This chapter has argued that embracing this approach will move the field closer to our common goal — to understand what therapists are doing that creates a significant impact, and to enhance the effectiveness of that process.

11

Behavior Therapy: Redefining Strengths and Limitations

By the end of the 1980s, a growing number of American psychologists involved in clinical and counseling activities identified themselves as behavior therapists or cognitive-behavior therapists (Mahoney, 1991). Although a large number of therapists are self-declared eclectics, many claim that cognitive-behavior therapy remains one of their major methods of intervention. Moreover, psychodynamic and experiential therapists alike have been pointing to the behavioral contributions to their own approaches (e.g., Anchin, 1987a; Barber & Luborsky, 1991; Bouchard & Derome, 1987; Greenberg, Safran, & Rice, 1989; Messer, 1986; Norcross, 1988; Reid, 1987; Wachtel, 1977). It seems fair to say, therefore, that a large percentage of psychotherapists have been directly or indirectly influenced by behavior therapy.

Having won recognition within the larger therapeutic community, behavior therapists have begun to evaluate their own shortcomings (e.g., Franks, 1984b; Mahoney, 1991). Whereas behavior therapy was once believed to be successful in nine out of ten cases (Wolpe, 1964), there is now a healthy recognition that our techniques have a more modest impact. Behavior therapy is now also more open about its failures and, much to its credit, has attempted to learn from them (Foa & Emmelkamp, 1983). All this points to a positive trend in behavior therapy's ongoing growth and development.

Despite its self-examination and self-criticism, behavior therapy has remained a major force in psychotherapy. By developing new assessment and treatment procedures, it has broken set with numerous traditions, and in doing so, has provided the field with undeniable contributions. But behavior therapy, like other therapeutic orientations, is imperfect. The intent of the present chapter is to highlight some of the strengths and limitations of the behavioral movement. For each of behavior therapy's contributions, it will be noted how these very strengths may also paradoxically serve to limit its clinical effectiveness. Although the focus is on cognitive-behavior therapy, it should not be concluded that all of these assets and liabilities are unique to this one orientation. Nor do we wish to foster a uniformity myth, implying that each strength and limitation of cognitive-behavior therapy reflects an asset or liability that inevitably exists in all clinical situations or disorders. Nonetheless, many of the general and rather global potential limitations of cognitive-behavior therapy have often followed from its strengths.

Consistent with the experimental roots of behavior therapy, its major contributions have been influenced by basic and applied research, as well as by the theoretical conceptualizations associated with these findings. A point that needs to be underscored, however, is that it has been our attempts as behavior therapists to *apply* conceptual and empirical contributions in clinical practice that have highlighted the shortcomings in cognitive-behavior therapy's strengths. Thus, the limitations may be more in the way we conceptualize and do research than in the way behavior therapy is actually practiced. Fortunately, new avenues are being explored within cognitive-behavior therapy in order to counteract some of its limitations. As will be pointed out, these avenues are often based on other theoretical orientations.

Strength #1: Behavior Therapy Characteristically Provides Us with a Fine-Grained Analysis of How Individuals React to Specific Life Situations

Reflecting its well-established experimental roots, behavior therapy approached complex and debilitating human problems by dimensionalizing them so that they could be thought of in terms of *variables*, which may be defined in very specific ways. Bandura's (1986) concept of "reciprocal determinism," for instance, has provided a fine-grained analysis of how behavioral, cognitive, and environmental variables are all mutually influential in understanding human functioning. At a clinical level, the focus on specific determinants of human behavior, rather than on global characteristics of clients, has opened new therapeutic avenues. Thus, instead of concluding that the fearful individual was "not ready to change," behavior therapists created hierarchies of increasingly more anxiety-producing situations that would allow for an ongoing progressive reduction in anxiety. This behavioral emphasis on specificity is much like looking at problematic reactions under a high-magnification microscope. We have encouraged a detailed examination of problematic thoughts, feelings, and behaviors in specific life situations, and a good deal of clinical and research effort has been devoted to developing both methods for the assessment of these molecular interactions and procedures for changing them.

Limitations. Even though this has clearly been one of behavior therapy's strengths, it may also result in a limitation. There is a trade-off involved when we engage in a microscopic analysis; the higher the magnification, the narrower the field of vision. Thus, one of the shortcomings of much of behavior therapy has been its failure to look at *patterns* of behavior—patterns that may span different times and settings in a client's life. This tradition of situational specificity may be readily traced to the early writings of Mischel (1968), described in Chapter 3, which established the behavioral view of personality as one that emphasized what people "did" in various situations, rather than what they "had" more globally. Disavowing such constructs as "traits," "needs," or "motives," Mischel (1969) went on to suggest that "what people do in any situation may be altered radically even by seemingly minor variations in prior experiences or slight modifications in stimulus attributes or in the specific characteristics of the evoking situation" (p. 1016).

In response to this argument against behavioral consistencies, Wachtel (1973) maintained that individuals who are likely to be seen in a clinical context almost by definition manifest behavior patterns that typically do not vary according to situation. Wachtel convincingly argued that it is precisely *because of* their failure to easily alter how they respond to situational changes that their functioning is impaired. It should be noted that in a later formulation of this issue, Mischel and Peake (1982) have suggested that although cross-situational consistency is unlikely, the temporal stability of an individual's prototypic characteristics may be found.

New directions. There are a number of ways in which we can become more sensitive to general patterns in our clients' lives. Wachtel (1977) has suggested that a psychodynamically oriented approach, particularly one that is interpersonal in emphasis, can be valuable in complementing behavior therapy by alerting it to the ways that individual interaction patterns may create problems in clients' lives. Also of relevance in this regard is the clinical–experimental work of Benjamin (1982), which characterizes reciprocal interpersonal relationship patterns along the dimensions of affiliation and control, as they occur both within and outside the context of therapy sessions. Focusing on the same dimensions of affiliation and control, Anchin (1987) has urged behavior therapists to incorporate several constructs and methods developed by interpersonal theorists within their empirical functional analysis of behavior. He argues that such expanded functional analyses would delineate important social factors that are generally disregarded in the current behavioral assessment of the antecedents, consequences, and nature of maladaptive behaviors.

The contributions of a systems approach, as reflected in current trends within behavioral marital therapy, may also be viewed as a move to alleviate the microscopic limitation within behavior therapy. By looking at more global patterns of marital interaction — like using a lower magnification microscope with a broader field — we can have a clearer picture of the overall context prior to our use of a fine-grain analysis of the relationship. Enlarging our focus of intervention by addressing the client's interpersonal system may also improve therapeutic effectiveness. A review of the relative merits of individual and/or marital interventions by Jacobson, Holtzworth-Munroe, and Schmaling (1989) has indicated that behavioral marital therapy is as effective as cognitive-behavior therapy for the treatment of depressive symptoms and, additionally, has a greater impact on marital satisfaction. As noted by Jacobson et al. (1989), considering the role of marital discord in precipitating and maintaining depression, the improvement of marital communication patterns might significantly reduce the client's relapse. In an attempt to capitalize on the potential synergistic effect of individual and marital interventions, Addis and Jacobson (1991) and Beach, Sandeen, and O'Leary (1990) have proposed theoretical and clinical guidelines to integrate cognitive-behavior therapy and behavioral marital therapy for the treatment of depression. As a function of social support and other possible factors, the involvement of the spouse in the treatment of agoraphobia seems to increase the therapeutic effect of behavioral exposure methods (Barlow, 1988). Jacobson et al. (1989) have underscored this point, also reporting studies suggesting that the addition of marital therapy to traditional outpatient treatment can provide an effective treatment for both alcohol-abuse problems and the marital difficulties that are implicated in these problems.

Although behavioral marital therapy addresses important elements of the client's interpersonal system (e.g., the couple's reciprocal use of punishments), its focus of intervention is still perceived by some cognitive-behavior therapists as too restrictive. Weiss (1980), for instance, has argued that by placing too much emphasis on the response or skill deficits of the partners (e.g., lack of positive reinforcers, communication-skills deficits), behavioral marital therapists have failed to consider the complex "dynamics" of the marital relationship (e.g., struggle for control, motivation to maintain relationship homeostasis). Such a narrow focus, according to Weiss, may account for problems of noncompliance observed in behavioral marital therapy. In order to deal with couple resistance to change, Weiss has elaborated a "Behavioral Systems Approach" that integrates strategic or systemic techniques (e.g., reframing, paradoxical intention, confusion) with the application of behavioral marital therapy.

Strength #2: Behavior Therapy Has Typically Been Dedicated to Development and Study of Specific Effective Techniques

As behavior therapists, we have at our disposal a wide array of different techniques that we can use when encountering different clinical problems. Because the methods are fairly well specified, they can be readily taught, researched, and perfected. From the early efforts with systematic desensitization and behavioral rehearsal to the more current work on exposure, communication training, and cognitive behavioral interventions, a considerable amount of clinical and research attention has been given to the development and study of different behavioral techniques. Cognitive-behavioral methods of intervention have been subjected to extensive research, and many have been demonstrated to be effective in treating various clinical problems. Here, too, behavior therapy can have two limitations in its strength, in that less attention has been paid to (a) individual client and therapist differences, and (b) the underlying principle of change. Each of these limitations is considered, in turn, below.

Limitation a: Individual differences.   With its emphasis on techniques, the behavior therapy literature may lead one to conclude that these methods can be adequately applied to all clients by all therapists. In this respect, cognitive-behavior therapy may have inadvertently contributed to maintaining one of the uniformity myths so aptly identified by Kiesler (1966). Consistent with the group comparison methodology that has characterized much of the outcome research on cognitive-behavior therapy, individual differences have been viewed as "error" or "noise." This tendency to neglect individual differences, as most clinicians well know, can readily undermine the effectiveness of our methods. The tacit assumption that individual differences play a relatively minor role may very well be the result of what we read in the research literature, where, for experimental purposes, subjects are randomly assigned to different treatment procedures. The clinical-research dichotomy is most evident here; we know of no clinical behavior therapist who randomly assigns a client to an intervention.

New directions.   This shortcoming has started to change, especially regarding the recognition of clients' individual differences along clinically meaningful dimensions. Clinical researchers, for example, are considering the interaction between the client's locus of control and the therapist's style of intervention. Thus, clients who need to be in control, a directive approach on the part of a therapist is likely to result in behavioral noncompliance (e.g., Beutler & Consoli, 1992; Shoham-Solomon, Avner, & Neeman, 1989). Beck (1983) has written about the sociotropic versus the autonomous client and the specific kinds of life situations that make them prone to depressive reactions. Karoly (1980) has described a number of individual differences in clients that may be relevant at various phases of the therapy process, from the recognition of a problem, to making a commitment to change, to the maintenance of change. Glass and Arnkoff (1982) have argued for matching cognitive-behavioral interventions with specific client styles of functioning (e.g., cognitive vs. action-oriented). Following this lead, attention to individual differences in the cognitive-behavioral treatment of anxiety disorders has begun to yield promising findings. For example, Michelson (1986) found that agoraphobic clients who received interventions that were designed to address their specific anxiety response profile (e.g., cognitive, behavioral, or physiological) improve more than those whose cognitive-behavioral interventions failed to address these individual differences. Preliminary findings by Nelson-Gray (1991) and her research group with unipolar depression similarly support the superiority of cognitive-behavioral interventions that match the response class associated with the specific client's depression (e.g., irrational beliefs, social skill deficits, infrequent pleasant activities).

Much less effort has been made to identify specific therapist factors that should guide the selection and administration of particular cognitive-behavioral interventions. This is noteworthy in light of research reviews pointing out the significant effect of certain therapist variables (e.g., personality, psychological adjustment) on client's improvement or deterioration (Crits-Cristoph et al., 1991; Lambert, 1989). An exception is the recent attention paid to the role of the therapist's personal reactions to the therapeutic relationship, which will be addressed in a later section of this chapter.

Limitation b: Overlooking principle of change. To the extent that cognitive-behavior therapists think in terms of techniques, they may also at times lose sight of the underlying principle of change reflected in the technique. The failure to look at the underlying principle can, in turn, prevent us from considering and experimenting with techniques that might be even more effective in implementing the change principle. Consider the clinical example of a 35-year-old female therapist. Although she seemed to be clinically competent, she was very unsure of her ability as a therapist, indicating that it had been several years since she worked in a clinical capacity. I suggested that perhaps what was needed was some practice, and urged her to sit in my chair and take the role of the therapist, talking to an imaginary client—a client who was very unsure about her ability to do therapy. She did a good job as therapist in this role-play situation and, in fact, was able to help herself in developing greater confidence in her ability to resume her work therapeutically. The question is, was this a behavioral role-playing technique that was used, or was it a gestalt two-chair exercise? My own view is that it is less relevant what we label our techniques, and more important that we identify their underlying principle of change. In the example given above, the important principle was to help the client obtain a more realistic vantage point on what she had been construing in a subjective and distorted way.

New directions.   Recent contributions have illustrated how techniques derived from different theoretical models can be used to implement the same strategies or processes of change (e.g., Goldfried, 1980a; Goldfried & Padawer, 1982; Prochaska & DiClemente, 1984). Moreover, this principle could probably be implemented by any of a number of different methods. Once psychotherapists start to think more in terms of principles of change, rather than in terms of the techniques prescribed by their preferred theory, they allow themselves the option of considering a far greater pool of intervention methods.

In nonbehavioral treatments, numerous clinical procedures have indeed been developed to implement different principles of change that are crucial to cognitive-behavior therapy, such as the facilitation of corrective experiences, ongoing reality testing, and, as mentioned above, the provision of a new perspective on self and the world (Brady et al., 1980). Consequently, we may well find that these intervention methods are not inconsistent with a cognitive-behavioral model of change, and can complement the behavior therapists clinical repertoire (cf. Lazarus, 1981). In addition, some of these interventions may be more effective than the cognitive-behavioral techniques we have developed for certain clinical problems. As suggested in Chapter 10, behavior therapists should consider using the two-chair gestalt technique when dealing with problematic choices in a client's life, as it has been shown to be more effective than problem-solving techniques (Clarke & Greenberg, 1986).

Strength #3: Behavior Therapy Makes Use of a Skill Training Orientation to Therapy

In rejecting the disease model of psychological problems, cognitive-behavior therapy has instead adopted an educational model, whereby clients are taught skills for coping with realistic life problems (Goldfried, 1980b). Thus, we serve not as healers, but rather as teachers, trainers, and consultants. As a reaction against early criticism that behavior therapy was undermining the client's autonomy and freedom of choice, behavior therapy developed a host of self-regulatory methods that could enable clients to function as their own therapists (Goldfried & Merbaum, 1973; Thoresen & Mahoney, 1974). Included among such coping methods have been relaxation, problem solving, cognitive restructuring, and interpersonal communication skills. Not only have these methods been useful within the clinical context, but they also have served as the bases for psychoeducational training programs, thereby reaching a broader population and having more far-reaching applications.

Limitation. Although this skill training emphasis has served us well in dealing with a number of clinical problems (e.g., unassertiveness), it may be limiting at times by fostering a tendency to lapse into a *didactic and overly directive approach* to intervention. In this regard, research findings by Patterson and Forgatch (1985) showed that therapeutic efforts at "teaching" parents to work more effectively with their children resulted in more noncompliance than did attempts at "support" and "facilitation." We have already alluded to the notion of noncompliance and how that is likely to occur with certain individuals for whom there is a high internal locus of control. A clinical example may serve to illustrate this point a bit more vividly.

Take the case of a 32-year-old, somewhat obsessional male high school teacher with a number of presenting problems. Should he marry? How well can he handle problems at work? How comfortable is he in social situations? He had been seen in the past by a number of other behavior therapists, all quite skilled. Although improvements were observed, changes never seemed to be maintained over time. In working with him clinically, I encountered the same problems; changes would occur, but they would not last. It was only after a while that I realized that my didactic approach to teaching assertion, relaxation, and other coping skills was, in fact, responsible not only for my own failure to bring about maintenance, but probably everyone else's as well. By being directive in teaching him coping skills, I was also inadvertently giving him the message that he *needed* directing, thereby unwittingly undermining his own self-efficacy. Once I became aware of the implicit message that was being conveyed by the nature of our therapeutic interaction, it provided a turning point in therapy. My strategy was to become very nondirective, on the assumption that he already had knowledge of and experience in the use of coping skills, and that his requests for direction and guidance, if satisfied, would only reinforce his lack of independence. Once the therapeutic relationship was based on a more nondirective footing, there was a very discernible positive change in his functioning.

New directions. Although cognitive-behavior therapy has described the importance of the collaborative relationship (e.g., Beck, Rush, Shaw, & Emery, 1979; Goldfried & Davison, 1976, 1994), it has been somewhat slow to recognize the inherent complexity and therapeutic value of the working therapeutic alliance (see Bordin, 1979). Emerging from a psychodynamic tradition, the construct of the working alliance has been shown to predict the client's improvement in cognitive-behavior therapy (see Gaston, 1990; Raue & Goldfried, 1994). Interestingly enough, a study of expert therapists (Raue, Castonguay, & Goldfried, 1993) found cognitive-behavior therapists to be rated significantly higher on the alliance than were psychodynamic therapists. Despite this unexpected finding, it may well be that cognitive-behavior therapists still have a lot to gain from the expertise of other therapists, especially when confronted with potential or actual strains in the therapeutic relationship. Safran, Crocker, McMain, and Murray (1990) have already illustrated the beneficial contributions to cognitive-behavior therapy from psychodynamic and humanistic orientations by defining specific signs of alliance strains (e.g., expression of negative feelings), as well as the use of several strategies to address such strains (e.g., awareness of one's own feelings; adopting an attitude of "participant-observer").

Systematic efforts to establish and maintain a therapeutic alliance have particularly been emphasized in the cognitive-behavioral approach to dealing with personality disorders. Linehan and her colleagues (Koerner & Linehan, 1992; Linehan, 1987), for example, have observed that challenging the irrational beliefs of borderline patients, or encouraging new ways of behaving, unwittingly serves to repeat the invalidating reactions of others that have painfully characterized their early social learning histories. By focusing on how borderline patients need to change, observes Linehan, the behavior therapist faces the danger of sending the latent message that they are deficient. Thus, the first strategy of her "dialectical behavior therapy" consists of establishing an accepting, empathic, and nondirective relationship. It is only after a strong working alliance has been secured with this patient population, and with their feeling that they have been fully accepted for just the way they are, that more traditional cognitive-behavioral techniques are implemented to help them acquire the coping skills that they generally lack.

Strength #4: Behavior Therapy Primarily Focuses on the Client's Current Life Situation

In behavioral interventions, the emphasis is on the "here and now" in the client's life, rather than the "there and then." In its attempt to avoid focusing on early childhood experiences—with the notable exception of dealing with issues of early abuse—cognitive-behavior therapy has dealt primarily with what is going on between sessions in the person's current life. The objective is to provide homework assignments, so that clients can take behavioral risks and have success experiences. As a result of this focus on between-session experiences, behavior therapy has been successful in shortening the course of interventions. However, it may also have kept it from paying sufficient attention to two other distinct arenas: (*a*) in-session issues and (*b*) the therapist's own reactions to the client. Each of these limitations is considered, in turn, below.

Limitation a: In-session issues.   Because of the focus on between-session problems or successes in the client's life, behavior therapy may at times overlook in-session issues, sometimes to the detriment of therapeutic progress. Take the example of the 51-year-old depressed accountant described in Chapter 9, who had a long history of previous psychodynamic therapy. It will be recalled that he entered cognitive-therapy because he wanted a more directive approach and something that would focus more on his current life situation. When assertiveness training was presented as a relevant approach in helping him to get better control over his current life and thereby alleviate his depression, the client responded with ambivalence. Although he wanted something that was different from what he had been doing in his past therapy, he continued to emphasize the need to get further insight into the developmental origins of his problem. I suggested, however, that the primary focus should be on encouraging more structured types of success experiences. The client agreed to the intervention procedures, but resisted following through on homework assignments. He also became increasingly more depressed, and indicated that he was not getting what he wanted from therapy. Precisely because he was so unassertive, he had difficulty in showing me his disappointment and anger directly. It was only after the focus was shifted to this in-session issue, and he was encouraged to express his anger toward me more directly, that he finally acknowledged that he could benefit from assertiveness training. From that point on, he became more cooperative in going out and asserting himself in various life situations and started to feel much more empowered in his interpersonal relationships.

New directions.   We noted earlier the importance of being mindful of how our directive interventions may at times lead to a client's noncompliance, as well as the need to maintain a good therapeutic alliance. The point to be made here, as suggested in earlier chapters, is that behavior therapy needs to acknowledge more generally that the therapeutic relationship can often provide us with a sample of the client's problem. That is, our interaction with clients can reflect a stimulus complex that at times may parallel the kinds of situations clients are having difficulty with outside the sessions. We hasten to add that it is not being suggested that the therapeutic relationship is always essential for providing the setting in which change occurs. On the other hand, clinical experience has convinced us that the client's reaction to the therapist as a significant other should at times be the essential focus of therapy. As psychodynamic authors have noted for close to a century, clients' emotional reactions to the therapist (such as hostility and ambivalence) provide important cues regarding how they interpret and react to others in their lives (Messer, 1986). Wright and Sabourin (1987) have similarly suggested that in behavior therapy, the exploration of client reactions (emotional, cognitive, and behavioral) toward the therapist can often lead to important benefits, such as the reduction of premature termination, the power struggle over homework assignments, or the minimization of clients' dependence at the end of the treatment.

The exploration of the client's reaction to the therapist has not been a preferred focus of intervention in behavior therapy, presumably because of the Freudian theoretical assumptions underlying the concept of "transference." However, several psychodynamic authors (e.g., Singer, 1988; Westen, 1988, 1991) have more recently reappraised the transference construct from the perspective of experimental cognitive psychology—an area to which some cognitive behavioral therapists have urged a close link (Goldfried & Robins, 1983; Mahoney, 1991). Despite behavior therapy's "phobia of transference" (Wright & Sabourin, 1987), systematic efforts have been undertaken by some behavior therapists to use the client's reaction toward the therapist for therapeutic purpose.

For example, Kohlenberg and Tsai (1989, 1991) have proposed a radical behavioral approach to therapy that places a primary focus on the therapeutic interaction. According to this view, the client's ways of relating to the therapist (e.g., being mad at the therapist for not knowing everything) represent *the* best possible source of observation of the client's difficulty, as well as the most salient and effective target of change. Reactions such as "intimacy difficulties, including fears of abandonment, rejection, engulfment; difficulties in expressing feelings; inappropriate affect, hostility, sensitivity to criticism" (Kohlenberg & Tsai, 1989, p. 391) are described as operants or respondents. Kohlenberg and Tsai maintain that such reactions are nonconsciously triggered by the therapeutic situations (i.e. controlling variables) because they have been learned from functionally similar interpersonal situations in the past (e.g., relationships with punitive and frustrating parents). The tasks of the therapist are to evoke, observe, reinforce, or extinguish the client's problems as they take place within the therapeutic session, to make the client aware of the functional relationship between the problematic behavior and the past and current environmental contingencies, and to provide the appropriate context to enable the client to learn more adaptive ways to behave. Although Kohlenberg and Tsai interpret the therapeutic relevance of these guidelines from conditioning models, one can hardly fail to see the parallels to psychodynamic theory.

In my own practice (see Chapter 9), I have found it useful to pay attention to clients' perception of and reaction to me, as well as to encourage them to express the feelings generated by my way of interacting with them. These "*in vivo*" interventions sometimes require a less active or directive attitude, forcing the therapist to maintain more of an observer's than a participant's role (Sullivan, 1954), so as to gain invaluable information about the clients' contributions to their current relational difficulties. These interventions also permit clients to learn that the expression of feelings to significant others does not necessarily lead to the disastrous consequences that they may have expected (cf. Alexander & French, 1946).

Limitation b: Our reactions to the client.   With behavior therapy's relative inattention to the therapeutic interaction, it also often failed to recognize the importance of the therapist's own reactions to the client. Henry, Schacht, and Strupp (1990) have shown that clients can evoke therapist hostility (i.e., blaming, ignoring, separating), especially in therapists who are critical toward themselves. Not surprisingly, such reactions were found to be associated with either no change or with actual deterioration. Although these findings were obtained in time-limited dynamic therapy, there is reason to believe that similar phenomena interfere with the conduct of cognitive-behavior therapy (Raue & Goldfried, 1994). As cogently observed by Wright and Sabourin (1987), "countertransference" may preclude behavior therapists from attending to important material, may increase the risk of inappropriate punishment, or may lead the therapist to impose treatment goals that may not be in the client's best interest.

New directions.   Several behavioral clinicians have recently attempted to demonstrate how the therapist's reaction to the client may serve important therapeutic purposes. As pointed out in Chapter 9, these reactions can provide invaluable information about how others in the client's day-to-day life may experience and respond to him or her. A similar observation was made by Kohlenberg and Tsai (1991), who have argued that from a radical behavioral viewpoint, the appropriate expression of the therapist's private reactions can function as a natural reinforcement for clients, and that the awareness of repeated strong negative (i.e., punitive) reactions should be used as an indication for referral. Other therapists working within the general framework of cognitive-behavior therapy have similarly begun to explore the use of self-disclosure to challenge clients' distorted perception of others (Arnkoff, 1983) and to prevent or address difficulties in the therapeutic alliance (Safran & Segal, 1990).

Strength #5: Behavior Therapy Has Been Influential in Encouraging Psychotherapy Outcome Research

Perhaps the most significant characteristic of behavior therapy, if not its *raison d'etre*, is a commitment to bridge the gap between scientific training and clinical practice (O'Leary & Wilson, 1987). By advocating an objective and controlled evaluation of treatment methods, behavior therapy not only has provided the field with effective and replicable techniques, but also has forced clinicians of other persuasions to demonstrate empirically their therapeutic effectiveness (cf. Eysenck, 1952). As shown in Gordon Paul's (1966) landmark study, behavior therapy has developed sophisticated experimental methodologies and, more importantly, has moved the field of behavior change to new directions of research — from the evaluation of the effectiveness of therapy in general to the study of specific interventions for targeted problems. Hence, for O'Leary and Wilson (1987), behavior therapy has brought about a scientific revolution:

> Behavior therapy has radically changed the nature of research on psychological treatment methods. Both the quantity and quality of studies on therapy outcomes have increased dramatically. Innovative research strategies allow rigorous evaluation of specific techniques applied to particular problems, in contrast to inadequate global assessments of poorly defined procedures applied to heterogeneous problems. (p. 11)

Limitation. The dedication of behavior therapy to the evaluation of psychological interventions has unquestionably been one of its most salient strengths (see O'Leary, 1984). Nonetheless, its scientific contribution has been primarily in the area of treatment outcome research. This emphasis has, in turn, tended to divert research energies away from *process research*, the focus of which is on studying the mechanisms of change. Consequently, although cognitive-behavior therapy has made significant strides in determining whether or not various behavioral procedures work, it has yet to acquire a clear understanding of how they work.

New directions. Process research is hardly a new direction in the field of psychotherapy. Therapy researchers primarily identified with psychodynamic or humanistic orientations have conducted an impressive number of studies on variables such as the clinicians' style, intentions, interpersonal skills, and involvement (Orlinsky & Howard, 1986). A wealth of empirical data has also been accumulated about clients' participation in therapy, such as their degree of engagement, initiative, openness, insight, conflict resolution, and emotional expressiveness (Elliott & James, 1989; Hill, 1990; Orlinsky & Howard, 1986).

Although process research has provided some substantive and reliable findings (see Orlinsky & Howard, 1986), it has not yet greatly advanced our understanding of therapeutic change (Rice & Greenberg, 1984). As cogently described by Strupp (1973a), early process studies have been conducted in a nonprogrammatic and isolated way. Moreover, some of the phenomena studied (e.g., frequency of the verbal occurrences) have failed to address the complexity of clinical reality and, therefore, remain removed from the real concerns of practitioners. Fortunately, a new generation of process researchers has emerged in recent years (Goldfried, Greenberg, & Marmar, 1990; Greenberg & Pinsof, 1986; Rice & Greenberg, 1984). They have developed innovative, yet rigorous research strategies (e.g., task analysis, interpersonal process recall, comprehensive process analysis; see Elliott, 1983; Elliott & James, 1989; Goldfried & Safran, 1986), with the goal of discovering important mechanisms of change in psychotherapy. Instead of focusing on the general issue of "therapy process"—including virtually anything that transpired between the therapist and client (e.g., duration of silences) — researchers are now looking more specifically at the "change process." Their methodologies are based on an intensive and contextual analysis of significant events that take place in different treatment phases. Still in its beginning stage, this new path of research has already led to the identification of recurrent therapist interventions and their impact on therapeutic change. Thus, Silberschatz, Fretter, and Curtis (1986) have shown that relative to theory-driven transference interpretations, therapists' interpretations that were specifically designed to deal with formulations of the patient's particular issues had more of an in-session impact.

With few exceptions (e.g., Goldfried, 1991; Schindler, Hohenberger-Sieber, & Hahlweg, 1989), cognitive-behavior therapists have not been involved in the development and application of these new research methodologies. Thus, although behaviorally-oriented researchers have been encouraged to study the effectiveness of other orientations (Wolfe, 1983), they may also be advised to consult psychodynamic and experiential therapy researchers on how to assess the significant patterns of interaction that may influence the outcome of their own interventions.

Strength #6: Behavior Therapy Has Provided Various Forms of Intervention to Reduce Specific Symptomatology

Rather than providing the same general approach to every type of psychosocial problem, cognitive-behavior therapy has developed a variety of interventions directly targeting the client's problem. Guided by the theoretical assumption that the "symptom is the neurosis," behavioral interventions have traditionally focused on the manifest problems (vs. hidden or latent cause) as felt by the client and/or as observed by others. Cognitive-behavioral methods are aimed at (1) emotions experienced as debilitating and uncontrollable (e.g., panic); (2) overt behaviors that the client wants to get rid of (e.g., compulsive rituals) or acquire (e.g., social skills); and (3) predominant and often explicit modes of thinking that interfere with functioning (e.g., catastrophic thinking). In doing so, cognitive-behavior therapy has made significant advances in developing methods for reducing the client's symptomatology.

Limitation. Because of the emphasis on treating problems that may best be characterized by Axis I disorders, behavior therapy has attended less to the *complexity of interpersonal problems* (e.g., personality disorders), instead dealing with explicit and isolated components of client functioning. And although the use of specific cognitive-behavioral methods in treating symptoms has unquestionably helped to advance the field, it soon became evident that attention needed to be refocused to personality disorders as well, as they were found to undermine the successful treatment of Axis I problems (Mavissakalian & Hamman, 1987; Rush & Shaw, 1983). Although originally wary of dealing with the construct of personality, behavior therapists—like Freud before them—have begun to move from symptomatic treatment to working with more complex personality issues (Lazarus, 1981).

New directions. In addressing the question of personality difficulties, a growing number of cognitive-behavior therapists have been inspired by the contributions of nonbehaviorists and have proposed new perspectives on how to conceptualize and treat emotional disorders. As mentioned previously, Linehan (1987) has underscored the importance of the therapist's empathic resonance in the treatment of borderline patients, acknowledging the relevance of Rogerian and Kohutian models of change. Safran and colleagues (Safran, 1990a, 1990b; Safran & Segal 1990), relying on the work of Sullivan, Kiesler, and Bowlby, have enriched cognitive-behavior therapists' concept of schema by integrating it with interpersonal and developmental perspectives. Knowledge of the teachings of gestalt therapy has also allowed them to highlight the role of affective processes in the development of psychopathology and adaptive human functioning. Based on the bridge that cognitive psychology has made between cognitive-behavior therapy and cognitively oriented psychodynamic therapy, R. Turner (1993) has developed a model of behavior therapy that incorporates dynamic thinking in dealing with a client's interpersonal problems.

Many of our cognitive behavioral theoretical assumptions have also been undergoing a redefinition by a group of therapists referred as "constructivists" (e.g., Guidano, 1990; Guidano & Liotti, 1983; Mahoney, 1991). Central to this redefinition is the belief in the individual's active participation in knowing and learning, the role of tacit processes in the perception of self and others, and the importance of emotional and interpersonal relationships throughout one's development. Guided by these assumptions, constructivists have developed treatments that focus on clients' history and unconscious knowing processes, and that recognize the importance of human subjectivity, intentionality, sense of identity, search for meaning, and the need for integrity. Constructivists' clinical practice is characterized by the expression and exploration of emotions, the acquisition of insights, and the establishment of a safe, caring, intense relationship that facilitates the exploration of self. Moreover, constructivists have emphasized the role of irrationality in human adaptation, the protective function of resistance, and the learning opportunities provided by relapse and regression (Mahoney, 1991).

Clinicians operating within the more traditional cognitive-behavioral framework have also been progressively more sensitive to the implicit intrapersonal and interpersonal aspects involved in severe psychological disorders (Beck, Freeman & Associates, 1990; Pretzer & Fleming, 1989; Young & Swift, 1988). Young and Swift (1988), for example, have identified tacit and enduring maladaptive schemas that may be at the roots of various personality disorders. These schemas, such as "defectiveness/unlovability" and "incompetence/failure," are believed to have resulted from dysfunctional relationship patterns during childhood. In Beck and associates' cognitive therapy for personality disorders, similar basic assumptions (e.g., "I am powerless and vulnerable," "I am inherently unacceptable") are the focus of the treatment, as well as the client's weak sense of identity. Among the clinical issues emphasized in this approach are the patient's "transference," difficulty with trust and intimacy, the therapist's frequent strong emotional reactions to the patient and need to set clear limits with regard to the patient's demands and behaviors (Beck et al., 1990).

In many respects, these recent efforts within cognitive-behavior therapy have begun to integrate some of the suggestions proposed by Messer (1986) regarding how we can benefit from psychodynamic therapy. For Messer, behavior therapy may find it helpful to foster the exploration, regulation, and integration of the client's inner reality (e.g., conflicts, emotions). Its clients may also benefit from an increased awareness of the origins of their problems in past conflictual relationships, thereby fostering the understandability of their irrational thoughts and schemas. Behavior therapists, according to Messer, may also overcome treatment resistance by being alert to the private reactions that emerge for both participants within the therapeutic interaction.

Like Messer, the point made in this and other chapters is that cognitive-behavior therapy could become more comprehensive, flexible, and ultimately more effective if it went beyond attempts to solely or immediately plan to reduce symptomatology, modify actions, and correct false beliefs. The helpfulness of other strategies and interventions will clearly have to be judged empirically. In the meantime, their theoretical and anecdotical support at least deserve serious consideration.

CONCLUSION

In noting the strengths and then highlighting the associated potential shortcomings of cognitive-behavior therapy, it would be misleading to conclude that it is worse off than are other orientations. Indeed, over the years, behavior therapy has developed a number of innovative, systematic procedures for dealings with a wide variety of clinical problems. Behavioral interventions have provided important break-throughs in the treatment of anxiety disorders, have given impetus to the development of the field of behavioral medicine, and have made inroads in the treatment of a variety of problems in children. In addition, the advocacy of methodological behaviorism has underscored the need to specify one's clinical methods and to subject them to empirical tests of accountability.

Not only have these tests confirmed that cognitive-behavior therapy can provide some powerful interventions for certain clinical problems, but they also have imposed new methodological standards on the field. Other orientations, particularly psychodynamic approaches to therapy, have been influenced by methodological behaviorism, as witnessed by the large number of therapy manuals involving short-term dynamic therapy that have been published (e.g., Klerman, Rounsaville, Chevron, & Weissman, 1984; Luborsky, 1984; Strupp & Binder, 1984). Experiential therapists have been less eager to submit their therapeutic claims to empirical verification. Despite the pioneering efforts of Rogers and his associates (see Mitchell, Bozarth, & Krauft, 1977; Truax & Mitchell, 1971), and with the more recent notable exceptions of Beutler and his colleagues (e.g., Beutler et al., 1991), Greenberg and his research group (e.g., Greenberg & Webster, 1982), and Mahrer and his associates (e.g., Mahrer & Nadler, 1986), there is relatively little in the way of research currently going on in this area. In fact, Wolfe (1983), of the National Institute of Mental Health, has announced that because there is a need for more empirical work on certain experiential procedures, behaviorally oriented researchers should be encouraged to apply for funding to study the effectiveness of such methods.

The clinical and methodological strengths of cognitive-behavior therapy, however, do not make it a "species" apart. All therapeutic orientations have limitations and blind spots. We have suggested that each of the unique strengths of the behavioral approach to therapy carries with it a potential concomitant weakness: Its fine-grained analysis of how individuals react to specific life situations has often tended to obscure the more general patterns of functioning within social systems. Its focus on developing and refining therapeutic techniques has caused it to attend less to individual client and therapist differences and general principles of change. Its adoption of an educational rather than a disease model, in which the emphasis is on teaching coping skills for dealing with life problems, has carried with it the risk of using an overly didactic and directive approach to intervention. Its emphasis on the client's ongoing, current life situation outside of therapy has diverted much of the attention away from potentially important issues within the therapy session itself. Its dedication to the demonstration of therapeutic efficacy through controlled outcome investigations has kept it from deploying it research efforts in process research. And its development of effective methods for reducing symptomatology has led many behavior therapists to pay less attention to the complexity of clients' interpersonal problems.

Recognizing such potential shortcomings can make us strong believers that cognitive-behavior therapists can learn from other approaches, even in the treatment of disorders for which they have come to be identified as the "experts." In the early 1980s, Barlow and Wolfe (1981) reported on the deliberation of a state-of-the-art conference on the behavioral management of anxiety disorders. With phobias, one of the types of problem with which behavior therapy is particularly effective, Barlow and Wolfe indicated that exposure procedures have been successful 75% of the time. However, if one takes into account those individuals who refuse to participate in the therapy, as well as those people who drop out prematurely, this rate shrinks to 49% (Barlow & Wolfe, 1981). Although some would argue that this success rate will increase as we continue to learn more about the parameters of exposure methods, a potentially more effective approach is to consider the possibility that perspectives based on other orientations may help behavior therapists assist their clients to accept the therapy that they offer, and to remain long enough in order to change. Clearly, this applies not only in the treatment of anxiety disorders, but also in the treatment of other types of clinical problems as well.

There is another important point that should be underscored. The strengths and concomitant potential limitations of cognitive-behavior therapy have, for the most part, been based on its theory and research findings. As students of behavior therapy all too well know, however, the theoretical and research literature does not always faithfully depict what goes on in clinical practice (cf. Goldfried & Davison, 1976, 1994; Lazarus & Davison, 1971). Our survey of cognitive-behavior therapists who all obtained their doctorates from the same university (Stony Brook) revealed the not too surprising finding that those who were primarily clinicians were more likely to have gone beyond the behavioral model than were those who worked within an academic setting (Friedling, Goldfried, & Stricker, 1984).

What practicing behavior therapists have known as part of their clinical "underground" (Wachtel, 1977) is now being fed back to create a reevaluation of the model as a whole. Such a reevaluation does not imply a repudiation of the basic empirical, conceptual, and clinical tenets of behavior therapy. We have argued elsewhere (Goldfried, Castonguay, & Safran, 1992) that the cognitive-behavioral approach, as well as the other major orientations, will probably continue their predominant positions in the future landscape of psychotherapy. Although behavior therapy will likely maintain its integrity and contact with its roots, its development may be enriched by incorporating theoretical and clinical contributions of other orientations.

SUMMARY

This chapter has highlighted some of the strengths and limitations that have been associated with the behavioral approach to intervention. For each of cognitive-behavior therapy's theoretical and empirical contributions, it was pointed out how these very strengths may also paradoxically serve to limit its clinical effectiveness. For the most part, the shortcomings in cognitive-behavior therapy's strengths have come to light as the result of attempts to apply these conceptual and empirical contributions in clinical practice. Included among the "limiting strengths" is the fact that behavior therapy has provided the field with a fine-grained analysis of how individuals react to specific life situations; has been dedicated to the development and study of specific effective techniques; makes use of a skill-training orientation to therapy; focuses on the client's current life situation; has been influential in encouraging psychotherapy outcome research; and has provided various forms of intervention to reduce specific symptomatology. Some of the new avenues, often based on other theoretical orientations, that are being explored by cognitive-behavior therapy in order to counteract some of its potential clinical limitations were also discussed.

Part V
THE CHALLENGE OF PSYCHOTHERAPY INTEGRATION

Behavior therapy is not the only orientation that has become interested in exploring the potential contributions of other theoretical frameworks. Psychodynamic thinkers, such as Wachtel (1977) have argued that psychodynamic interventions could benefit considerably by incorporating certain behavioral procedures. The strong adversarial stance that had been taken by different therapy orientations has softened considerable during the 1980s. And even though the different social systems that have comprised the field of psychotherapy have typically been oppositional and seemingly mutually exclusive, there has always been a tendency for practicing clinicians to step out of the conceptual constraints that may characterize their orientation. Indeed, this was noted by the late Perry London back in the 1960s, when discussing limitations associated with either a pure form psychodynamic or behavioral orientation:

> There is a quiet blending of techniques by artful therapists of either school; a blending that takes account of the fact that people are considerably simpler than the Insight schools give them credit for, but that they are also more complicated than the Action therapists would like to believe. (London, 1964, p. 39)

Over the years, there have been scattered attempts to bridge the gaps between different therapy orientations. As described in Chapter 12, a very early example can be traced to the 1932 meeting of the American Psychiatric Association, where Thomas French delivered an address in which he attempted to draw parallels between psychoanaly-

181

tic thinking and Pavlovian conditioning. This chapter traces the 50-year history of psychotherapy integration from French's noteworthy presentation until the early 1980s.

Even though therapists from varying orientations were writing about what they believed to be the active ingredients to therapeutic change from within their own particular framework, a careful reading of the literature reveals some interesting commonalities. For example, in the same year I published the original article outlining rational restructuring as a self-control technique (Goldfried, Decenteceo, & Weinberg, 1974), Bieber (1974) described a remarkably similar therapeutic strategy that could be used within a psychoanalytic context. Moreover, Rice (1980) quite independently developed a similar intervention from within her own, client-centered orientation.

Chapter 13 describes a conceptual model for uncovering commonalities across different theoretical orientations. Based on the writings of therapists from behavioral, psychodynamic, and experiential orientations, I suggest that common factors in the change process may be looked at from a level of abstraction somewhere between the specific techniques and the more general theory used to explain why the techniques may work. It is at this level of the clinical strategy that common, indeed, robust principles of change may be revealed.

Some of these common principles are outlined in Chapter 14, including the therapeutic benefit clients may experience from having expectations that therapy will be helpful; participating in an optimal therapeutic relationship; obtaining a more realistic perspective on themselves and their world; having corrective experiences; and being provided with the opportunity to repeatedly test current reality. Although this chapter argues for the importance of looking at common factors, it also acknowledges some of the unique contributions that the psychodynamic, behavioral, and experiential traditions have brought to the therapeutic enterprise. Moreover, it underscores the importance of having a supportive professional network to explore psychotherapy integration, and outlines the steps that were used to form SEPI—the Society for the Exploration of Psychotherapy Integration.

Moving from what was a latent theme dating back to the early 1930s, and more recently having developed into a definite movement, psychotherapy integration has clearly made an important mark on the field of psychotherapy. If nothing else, it has raised the consciousness of therapists of different orientations, apprising them of both similarities across orientations as well as the unique contributions that another orientation might make to their own. The question of what the future holds in store and where we need to go in order to advance the psychotherapy integration movement is addressed in Chapter 15. Taken from an article written with Louis Castonguay, this chapter makes the argument that it would be unrealistic to expect any revolutionary changes in the field of psychotherapy as a result of work in psychotherapy integration. More likely, there is apt to be an evolutionary change, where therapists will be open to whatever they can use to enhance their clinical effectiveness, regardless of its theoretical roots. Indeed, the threats from outside the field of psychotherapy—biological psychiatry and managed health care—provide a significant impetus for therapists to move in this direction.

12

On the History of
Therapeutic Integration

The idea of being able to integrate varying approaches to psychotherapy has intrigued mental health professionals for some time. Only since the 1980s, however, has the issue of rapprochement developed into a more clearly delineated "area of interest." Prior to that time, it was more of a latent theme that ran through the psychotherapy literature. The topic of rapprochement has rarely been indexed in any bibliographic sources, making the task of carrying out an historical analysis somewhat difficult. A fair amount of the relevant literature came to light through citations made by other authors in pertinent articles, chapters, and books. Inasmuch as references are still continuing to emerge, it is safe to say that the review is far from complete, and a more comprehensive review may be found elsewhere (Goldfried & Newman, 1992).

The hope of finding some consensus across the psychotherapies can be traced back to the early 1930s. It should be noted that it is not always easy to determine the precise impact that earlier trends may have had on later thinking. Even if an idea is rejected outright, it cannot be assumed that it has made no impact. If nothing else, it probably has served a consciousness-raising function, in that it called the field's attention to a particular issue. Perhaps, as Kendall (1982) suggests, the field must reach a certain level of development before it can seriously entertain certain notions. The present chapter highlights the trends toward rapprochement, and comments more generally on the task of achieving an integration among the psychotherapies.

EARLY ATTEMPTS AT INTEGRATION

In perhaps what represented one of the earliest attempts at integrating the psychotherapies, French delivered an address at the 1932 meeting of the American Psychiatric Association, in which he drew certain parallels between psychoanalysis and Pavlovian conditioning. Acknowledging the wide discrepancy between these two approaches, French discussed the similarities between the psychoanalytic concept of repression and Pavlovian concepts of extinction and inhibition. Trying to tie sublimation to learning principles, he invoked the principle of differentiation, suggesting that some sort of discrimination training had probably taken place to differentiate the unacceptable from the more socially accepted manifestations of certain impulses. He also suggested that a patient's adjustment to reality might be explained in terms of the individual's earlier conditioned experiences.

The text of French's presentation was published in the following year (French, 1933), along with comments from members of the audience. As one might expect, French's presentation resulted in very mixed audience reaction. In one of the most unabashedly negative responses by a member of the audience, Myerson acknowledged:

> I was tempted to call for a bell-boy and ask him to page John B. Watson, Ivan Pavlov, and Sigmund Freud, while Dr. French was reading his paper. I think Pavlov would have exploded; and what would have happened to Watson is scandalous to contemplate, since the whole of his behavioristic school is founded on the conditioned reflex . . . . Freud . . . would be scandalized by such a rapprochement made by one of his pupils, reading a paper of this kind. (In French, 1933, p. 1201)

Adolf Meyer was not nearly as unsympathetic. Although stating that the field should encourage separate lines of inquiry, and not attempt to substitute any one for another too prematurely, Meyer nonetheless suggested that one should "enjoy the convergencies which show in such discussions as we have had this morning" (in French, 1933, p. 1201). Gregory Zilboorg, who was also in the audience at the time, took an even more favorable stand, noting:

> I do not believe that these two lines of investigation could be passed over very lightly . . . . There is here an attempt to point out, regardless of structure and gross pathology, that while dealing with extremely

complex functional units both in the physiological laboratory and in the clinic, we can yet reduce them to comparatively simple phenomena. (In French, 1933, pp. 1198–1199)

In an extension of French's attempts, Kubie (1934) maintained that certain aspects of psychoanalytic technique itself could be explained in terms of the conditioned reflex. Noting that Pavlov hypothesized that certain associations might exist outside of an individual's awareness because they took place under a state of inhibition, Kubie suggested that the encouragement of free association on the part of the patient, and the relatively passive role of the therapist, might serve to remove the conditions of inhibition and thus allow such unconscious associations to emerge into conscious awareness.

In 1936, Rosenzweig published a brief article in which he described what he believed were common factors among the psychotherapies. In contrast to French's and Kubie's attempts to link two separate theoretical orientations, Rosenzweig argued that the effectiveness of various therapeutic approaches probably had more to do with their common elements than with the theoretical explanations on which they were based. Rosenzweig suggested three common factors: (a) Regardless of any particular orientation one adopts, it is the personality of therapists themselves that have much to do with the effectiveness of the change process, perhaps related to their ability to inspire hope in patients or clients. (b) Interpretations that therapists might make to patients are helpful because they provide an alternative and perhaps more plausible way of understanding one's problem. It makes little difference what the interpretation is, argued Rosenzweig, as long as it serves to make one's problem more understandable. (c) Even though varying theoretical orientations may focus on different aspects of human functioning, they can all be effective because of the synergistic effects that one area of functioning might have on another.

At the 1940 meeting of the American Orthopsychiatric Association (Watson, 1940), a small group of therapists got together to discuss areas of agreement in psychotherapy. Commenting on the points of commonality (e.g., the importance of the therapeutic interaction), Watson observed that ". . . if we were to apply to our colleagues the distinction, so important with patients, between what they tell us and what they do, we might find that agreement is greater in practice than in theory" (p. 708).

The next major work in the history of the integration of the psychotherapies consisted of Dollard and Miller's classic book *Personality and Psychotherapy*, published in 1950 and dedicated to "Freud and Pavlov and their students." The importance of Dollard and Miller's work in the history of psychotherapy can be attested to by the fact that this book was continually in print for over 30 years. Although behavior therapists have traditionally argued that Dollard and Miller's thinking had little impact on the development of behavior therapy, such repeated references to this work would certainly suggest that the book was widely read. In their work, Dollard and Miller described in detail how such psychoanalytic concepts as regression, anxiety, repression, and displacement might be understood within the framework of learning theory. For the most part, Dollard and Miller only translated one language system into another. Nonetheless, they did point to certain factors that may very well be common to all therapeutic approaches, such as the need for the therapist to support an individual's attempt at changing by expressing empathy, interest, and approval for such attempts.

Even though Dollard and Miller (1950) stayed fairly close to the intervention procedures associated with psychoanalytic therapy, they made continual reference to principles and procedures on which contemporary behavior therapy is based. Thus, Dollard and Miller suggest the value of modeling procedures (e.g., "watching a demonstration of the correct response may enable the student to perform perfectly on the first trial," pp. 37–38); the use of hierarchically arranged tasks (e.g., "the ideal of the therapist is to set up a series of graded situations where the patient can learn." p. 350); reinforcement of gradual approximations toward a goal (e.g., "if a long and complex habit must be learned, the therapist should reward the subunits of the habit as they occur." p. 350); the principle of reciprocal inhibition, (e.g., "like any other response, fear apparently can be inhibited by responses that are incompatible with it." p. 74); the significance of the reinforcing characteristics of the therapist (e.g., "the therapist uses approval to reward good efforts on the part of the patient." p. 395); the emphasis on between-session assignments (e.g., "behavioral changes must be made in the real world of the patient's current life. If benevolent changes are to occur, the patient must begin doing something new." p. 319); the importance of teaching the individual self-control or coping skills to be used following therapy (e.g., "it is theoretically possible that special practice in self-study might be given during the latter part of a course of therapeutic interviews. The patient might be asked to practice solving particular problems . . . [under conditions] as similar as possible as those to be used after therapy," p. 438); the treatment of orgasmic dysfunctions via masturbation (e.g., "at one point in a therapeutic sequence, the therapist might have to reward masturbation so that the patients may experience the sexual orgasm for the first time." p. 350); and the importance of environmental contingencies for maintaining behavior change (e.g., "the conditions of real life must be favorable if new responses are to become strong habits." p. 427).

Unlike Dollard and Miller (1950), whose primary emphasis was on the integration of different theoretical orientations, Thorne (1950) was interested in pursuing therapeutic integration on the basis of what we know empirically about how people function and change. Thorne's book on eclectic psychotherapy (*Principles of Personality Counseling*) was based on some of his work published in the *Journal of Clinical Psychology*, which he founded 5 years earlier. From the time that he was a medical student, Thorne was struck by the fact that medicine was not divided up into different schools of thought, but rather that basic principles of bodily functioning were what guided actual practice. One objective throughout his career was to establish a similar set of principles for the field of psychology and psychotherapy. Garfield (1957), who similarly has long been interested in an empirically based approach to therapy, outlined what appeared to be common points among the psychotherapies. In this introductory clinical psychology text, Garfield noted such universal factors as an understanding and supportive therapist, the opportunity for emotional catharsis, and the provision of self-understanding.

MORE RECENT TRENDS TOWARD RAPPROCHEMENT

Little, if anything else, was written about therapeutic rapprochement until the early 1960s. Perhaps it was the conservative social and political climate of the 1950s that served to discourage therapists from questioning their paradigm. Whatever the reason, the next decade witnessed an increasing number of books and articles dealing with rapprochement.

1960s

The most significant contribution to the integration of the psychotherapies appearing in the early 1960s came with the publication of Frank's (1961) *Persuasion and Healing*. This book addresses itself to commonalities cutting across varying attempts at personal influence. Frank suggested that psychotherapy served to correct misconceptions that individuals have about themselves and others. However, psychotherapy was not the only method for influencing people, observed Frank; similar change processes could be seen in such diverse methods as religious conversion, primitive healing, brainwashing, and the placebo effects that occur in the practice of medicine. When distressed individuals are placed in any of these contexts, the effectiveness of the interaction involves some expectancy for improvement and an arousal of hope, eventually resulting in a concomitant increase in self-esteem and improved functioning. Although Frank continued to be an advocate of common factors across the psychotherapies in his later writings, one of his later reviews of the current status of the field (Frank, 1979) acknowledged that certain clinical problems (e.g., fears, phobias, compulsive rituals) may be effectively dealt with by methods that go beyond the general nature of the therapeutic interaction.

In one of the last papers to be published before his death, Alexander (1963), a colleague of French, suggested that psychoanalytic therapy might profitably be understood in terms of learning theory. On the basis of an analysis of tape recordings made of psychoanalytic therapy sessions, Alexander came to the conclusion that many of the changes that occurred therapeutically "can best be understood in terms of learning theory. Particularly the principle of reward and punishment and also the influence of repetitive experiences can be clearly recognized" (p. 446). As a therapist who was dedicated to the advancement of the field throughout his career, Alexander suggested "We are witnessing the beginnings of a most promising integration of psychoanalytic theory with learning theory, which may lead to unpredictable advances in the theory and practice of the psychotherapies."

(p. 448). Also as an outgrowth of the same program of research on psychotherapy in which Alexander was involved, Marmor (1964) described in detail the learning principles that he believed to underlie psychoanalytic therapy.

In the same year that Alexander's paper appeared, Carl Rogers (1963) published an article dealing with the current status of psychotherapy. He noted that the field was "in a mess," but that the theoretical orientations within which therapists had typically functioned were starting to break down. He stated that the field was now ready to shed itself of the limitations inherent in specific orientations—including client-centered therapy—and that we needed to observe more directly exactly what goes on during the course of psychotherapy.

London (1964), in a short but insightful book entitled *The Modes and Morals of Psychotherapy*, pointed to the inherent limitations associated with both the psychodynamic and behavioral orientations, suggesting:

> There is a quiet blending of techniques by artful therapists of either school; a blending that takes account of the fact that people are considerably simpler than the Insight schools give them credit for, but that they are also more complicated than the Action therapists would like to believe. (p. 39)

Marks and Gelder (1966) also compared behavior therapy and psychodynamic procedures, looking at their historical antecedents, theoretical underpinnings, practical procedures, and claims to success. Although acknowledging that there was probably common ground between the two approaches, Marks and Gelder also underscored certain differences. They further suggested that the two approaches should be viewed as potentially contributing to each other, rather than necessarily being antagonistic in nature. Arguing for the integration of learning theory with psychoanalysis, Wolf (1966) noted:

> I submit that their integration is sooner or later inevitable, however passionately some or many of us may choose to resist it. Psychoanalysis cannot remain for much longer outside the behavioral sciences, nor can the science of human behavior for much longer ignore the body of knowledge amassed by the psychoanalytic schools of thought. (p. 535)

The concept of "technical eclecticism" was introduced in 1967 by Lazarus, who maintained that techniques from various therapeutic systems may be used by clinicians without necessarily accepting the theoretical underpinnings associated with these methods. Starting from this pragmatic/clinical point of view, Lazarus suggested that the ultimate standard of utility should rest on empirical, not theoretical grounds. Appearing in that same year was an article by Patterson (1967) on divergent and convergent elements across the psychotherapies, and also a paper by Whitehouse (1967) in *Rehabilitation Literature*, in which he discussed generic principles underlying a wide variety of therapeutic interventions.

Brady (1968), responding to the practical demands of doing actual clinical work, argued that behavioral and psychodynamic approaches were not necessarily contradictory in nature, but could be used in combination with certain cases. He described the treatment of a preorgasmic woman who experienced anxiety associated with sexual activities, where successful treatment was accomplished by means of systematic desensitization and short term psychodynamic therapy focusing on her relationship with her husband. Leventhal (1968) similarly described a case of a patient experiencing anxiety over sexuality who was successfully treated with a combined behavioral and traditional therapeutic intervention. In an article offering a rationale for "psychobehavioral therapy," Woody (1968) maintained that the integration of behavior therapy and psychodynamic therapy was particularly relevant for cases that were unresponsive to treatment.

In a theoretical paper examining the similarities among psychoanalytic, behavioral, and client-centered therapy, Sloane (1969) maintained that common factors ran through all three orientations. Sloane suggested that, in the final analysis, the underlying process associated with therapeutic change probably involves learning principles. In a commentary on Sloane's paper, Marmor (1969) agreed that all therapies involve some application of learning principles, either directly or unwittingly, but did not believe that the simple S-R model could explain some of the more complex aspects of human functioning. Moreover, like London (1964), Marks and Gelder (1966), Lazarus (1967), Brady (1968), and others, Marmor concluded that behavioral and psychodynamic therapies are probably best viewed as complementary in nature, with neither model being totally applicable to all cases. Cautioning against a haphazard piecing together or techniques from different orientations, Brammer (1969) maintained that the type of eclecticism the field needed was one based on research findings on the effectiveness of various clinical procedures.

1970s

Birk (1970), writing in the newly formed journal *Behavior Therapy*, described two clinical cases to illustrate the potential integration of behavior therapy with psychodynamic theory. Commenting on how existing cultural values contribute to the development of different schools of therapy, Frank (1971) outlined features that nonetheless were common to all approaches. Marmor published an article on therapeutic integration in that same year (Marmor, 1971), in which he suggested:

> The research on the nature of the psychotherapeutic process in which I participated with Franz Alexander, beginning in 1958, has convinced me that all psychotherapy, regardless of the techniques used, is a learning process . . . . Dynamic psychotherapies and behavior therapies simply represent different teaching techniques, and their differences are based in part on differences in their goals and in part on their assumptions of the nature of psychopathology. (p. 26)

Marmor's clinical observation that cognitive learning occurs during the course of therapy in addition to simple conditioning is probably a conclusion with which many contemporary behavior therapists would now agree.

In a comprehensive and scholarly review of the psychotherapy outcome literature, Bergin (1971) recognized the important empirical contributions that behavior therapy had begun to make. Nonetheless, he concluded that the field needed to remain open to the "many fertile leads yet to be extracted from traditional therapy" (p. 254). Responding to his clinical observations that behavior therapy alone was not always effective clinically, Lazarus (1971) described in *Behavior Therapy and Beyond* a wide array of both behavioral and nonbehavioral techniques that may be employed by broad-spectrum behavior therapists. In the same year, Woody (1971) also published a book integrating behavioral and insight-oriented procedures. Echoing Lazarus's concept of technical eclecticism, Woody suggested that, providing one is able to set aside varying theoretical allegiances, the practicing clinician is capable of selecting and integrating procedures from varying sources based purely on pragmatic grounds. Marks (1971) similarly noted the beginning trends toward rapprochement, observing that therapists "are growing less reluctant to adopt methods and pedigrees outside their own theoretical systems" (p. 69).

Houts and Serber's (1972) edited book *After the Turn-on, What?* described the experiences of a group of seven researchers and practitioners who spent a weekend together participating in a humanistic group-type experience. Ranging from radical behavioristic to cognitive learning in orientation, the participants described what they saw to be both assets and liabilities of their group experience. As a part of a larger project to try to determine the future course of psychotherapy research, Bergin and Strupp (1972) reported on their contacts with researchers throughout the country. Among those who were interviewed was Neal Miller, who predicted that as behavior therapy began to become involved with more complicated types of cases, and as psychodynamic therapy focused more on ego mechanisms and the working through process, the two therapeutic approaches would eventually start to converge in some interesting ways. In a provocative article dealing with the "end of ideology" in behavior therapy, London (1972) asked his behavioral colleagues to call a truce in their strife with other orientations and to look more realistically and pragmatically at what we are able to do clinically. Very much the clinical pragmatist, London cautioned us against becoming overly enamored with our theories of therapy, noting: "The first issue, scientifically as well as clinically, is the factual one — do they work? On whom? When? The how and why come later" (p. 919). And if techniques exist that are not necessarily within the behavioral school but are found to be effective, continued London, these cannot afford to be ignored. Other attempts at therapeutic integration that appeared in 1972 included a book by Martin that attempted to integrate learning theory with client-centered therapy, a set of two papers dealing with the theoretical and clinical aspects associated with the integration of psychodynamic and behavior therapies (Feather & Rhoads, 1972a, 1972b), and a description of universal healing processes, seen among psychotherapists and witchdoctors alike (Torrey, 1972).

Commenting on one of the Feather and Rhoads articles appearing in the previous year, Birk (1973) noted that one area of complementarity between a behavioral and psychodynamic approach was that the former dealt more with external stimuli, whereas the latter tended to focus on stimuli that were more internal in nature. Strupp (1973b), dealing more with the common elements underlying all psychotherapies, underscored the therapeutic relationship as a vehicle for change, providing the client/patient with corrective learning experiences. Strupp likened the therapeutic interaction to a parent–child relationship, a phenomenon that Freud had called "after-education." In a chapter entitled "Behavioral Humanism," Thoresen (1973) suggested that many of the philosophical underpinnings associated with these two orientations were in agreement, and that it was possible to view a behavioral approach as providing the technology by which certain humanistic goals might be achieved. Also appearing in that same year was a report of two cases treated for sexual deviance (Woody, 1973), in which successful treatment was accomplished by aversion therapy and short term psychodynamic therapy, administered concurrently by separate therapists.

Quite a bit was written in 1974 on the issue of therapeutic rapprochement. In an intriguing article that described behavioral and psychodynamic approaches as "complementary" rather than mutually exclusive, Ferster (1974)—a former student and colleague of Skinner—presented what he observed to be some of the merits of psychoanalytically oriented therapy. Birk and Brinkley-Birk (1974) provided a conceptual integration of psychoanalysis and behavior therapy, viewing the two approaches as complementing "the weak links in the therapeutic input-outcome chain of the other" (p. 505). They specifically suggested that with an integrated model, insight can set the stage for change, whereas behavior therapy provides some of the actual procedures by which the change process may be brought about. They went on to suggest that: "What is really required at this stage, however, is a dialogue between clinicians of both schools whose aim is genuine rapprochement, mutual understanding, and the tentative forging of a new clinical learning theory for psychotherapy." (p. 500). Birk (1974) illustrated how intensive group therapy might be implemented by combining behavioral and psychoanalytic principles, and Rhoads and Feather (1974) described cases that were treated with desensitization procedures that were modified along psychodynamic lines.

Kaplan (1974), in her book *The New Sex Therapy*, outlined how a psychodynamic approach to therapy may be integrated with performance-based methods. In a report of the Menninger Foundation Psychotherapy Research Project, Horwitz (1974, 1976) noted that inasmuch as supportive treatment procedures produced just as effective outcomes as insight-oriented therapy, the psychodynamic approach needed to consider alternate methods of producing therapeutic change that might not readily fit into its usual conceptual model. Silverman (1974) similarly made suggestions to his psychoanalytic colleagues that there is much to learn from "other approaches" that can make (unmodified) psychoanalytic treatment more effective" (p. 305). In a paper delivered at the 1974 meeting of the American Psychological Association, Landsman urged his humanistically oriented colleagues to attend to some of the important contributions of behavior therapy, such as "attention to specifics, to details, careful quantification, modesty in claims, demonstrable results" (p. 15).

In his book *Misunderstandings of the Self*, Raimy (1975), like Frank (1961), suggested that various approaches to therapy all seem to be directed toward changing clients' misconceptions of themselves and of others. All therapies are alike in that they "present evidence" to assist individuals in changing these misconceptions, but that the type of evidence and the way that it is presented varies across different therapeutic orientations. In Egan's (1975) clinically oriented book on the therapeutic change process, he modified his original humanistic orientation to acknowledge that there comes a time when the therapist must assume a more active role in helping a client to change. Although the contributions of Rogers (1963) and others are essential for establishing the type of therapeutic relationship in which change can take place, Egan suggested that behavior therapy may offer the clinician methods to implement specific action programs.

Referring to the contributions made by Alexander, Horney, and Sullivan to psychodynamic therapy, Wachtel (1975) maintained that behavioral approaches, which attempt to deal directly with certain problematic behaviors, can readily be incorporated into a psychodynamic framework. This is a two-way street, argued Wachtel, in that many instances of relapse following behavior therapy might possibly be linked to certain maladaptive patterns on the part of the patient. These patterns in turn might more readily be identified when viewed from within a psychodynamic framework. Wachtel (1977) went on to explore such integration at greater length in his thought-provoking book *Psychoanalysis and Behavior Therapy*, in which he maintained that the convergence of clinical procedures from each orientation would be likely to enhance the effectiveness of our intervention attempts. For example, a psychodynamic orientation might help us to better understand the implicit meaning structures and distortions that our clients carry with them in their current life situation, whereas the behavioral approach could provide us with techniques by which we may actively intervene in changing such distortions. Focusing on a more theoretical level, Shectman (1975) suggested that behavioral principles might provide psychoanalysis with a more adequate theory of learning.

The year 1976 also witnessed a number of articles and books that touched on the topic of therapeutic integration. Strupp (1976) criticized psychoanalytic therapy for not keeping up with the times, using therapeutic procedures more on the basis of faith than data. Fortunately, observed Strupp, younger therapists appear to be less constrained by orthodoxy, and are more willing to experiment with newer techniques. In a commentary on Strupp's article, Grinker (1976) underscored the need for a therapeutic approach based on research findings and noted that with added clinical experience, even the most orthodox of psychoanalysts learn that other methods are needed to help facilitate change. As a practicing psychoanalyst who had personal experience with the human potential movement, Appelbaum (1976) suggested that some of the methods of gestalt therapy may complement more traditional psychoanalytic techniques. Appelbaum's excursions into more humanistically oriented activities are described in fascinating detail in a later book of his (Appelbaum, 1979).

Wandersman, Poppen, and Ricks's (1976) *Humanism and Behaviorism* provided a collection of chapters by members of each orientation, in which there was an attempt to acknowledge points of potential integration. Burton's (1976) edited volume *What Makes Behavior Change Possible?* contained chapters by 16 representatives of a wide diversity of therapeutic orientations, all of whom addressed themselves to some of the basic questions associated with the essential ingredients of therapeutic change. Noting that behavior therapy was a useful framework for dealing with clinical cases, but still incomplete in and of itself, Hunt (1976) argued that there currently exists no single orientation that can deal with all clinical material. Just as separate laser beams function together to obtain a three-dimensional holographic image, observed Hunt, so are different therapeutic orientations required in order to provide us with a comprehensive treatment approach.

In their book *Clinical Behavior Therapy*, Goldfried and Davison (1976) maintained that behavior therapy need no longer assume an antagonistic stance vis-à-vis other orientations. Acknowledging that there is much that clinicians of different orientations have to say to each other, they suggested that it was time for behavior therapists to enter into dialogues with their nonbehavioral colleagues. That many clinicians were in effect already doing this was reflected in Garfield and Kurtz's (1976) findings that approximately 55% of clinical psychologists in the United States considered themselves to be eclectic. The two most frequent orientations used in combination were psychodynamic and learning. The single most frequent reason for using more than one framework was found to be based on the pragmatics of doing clinic work (Garfield & Kurtz, 1977). This integration at a clinical level was dealt with in several articles (Lambley 1976; Levay, Weissberg, & Blaustein, 1976: Murray, 1976; Segraves & Smith, 1976). Also, Lazarus's (1976), *Multimodel Behavior Therapy*, extended and refined his broad-spectrum approach to behavior therapy so as to systematically take into account the individual's behavior, affect, sensations, images, cognitions, interpersonal relationships, and physiological states.

In the following year, Lazarus (1977), then having practiced behavior therapy for approximately 20 years, questioned the possibility that behavior therapy as a delimited school of thought had "outlived its usefulness." He recognized the need to "transcend the constraints of factionalism, where cloistered adherents of rival schools, movements, and systems each cling to their separate illusions" (p. 11). Also, Lazarus reiterated his earlier statement on technical eclecticism, suggesting that empirically determined effectiveness and not therapeutic school should dictate what intervention procedures we use.

An editorial comment appearing in the *Journal of Humanistic Psychology* (Greening, 1978) applauded Lazarus's 1977 paper, urging the readership of the Journal to be open to such suggestions for rapprochement. Commenting on the gap that frequently exists between theory and practice, Davison (1978) delivered a presentation at the Association for Advancement of Behavior Therapy (AABT) Convention in which he suggested that behavior therapists consider the possibility of using certain humanistic procedures in their clinical work. Krasner (1978) outlined the history of both behaviorism and humanism, noting that both orientations shared some common views of human functioning (e.g., importance of situational factors, the uniqueness of the individual). He looked forward to the time when representatives in "both camps will decrease mutual battling and recriminations and join against a common foe and, most important, for a mutual goal" (p. 803). In that same year, Baer and Stolz (1978) provided a behavioral analysis of *est*, and O'Leary and Turkewitz (1978) described how a communication analysis of marital interaction might be used within the context of behavioral marital therapy. Some of the points of overlap between behavior therapy and Zen Buddhism were outlined by Mikulas (1978) and Shapiro (1978).

A symposium on the compatability and incompatibility of behavior therapy and psychoanalysis, chaired by Arkowitz, was held at the 1978 AABT Convention. In an independent convention paper entitled "Are Psychoanalytic Therapists Beginning to Practice Cognitive Behavior Therapy or is Behavior Therapy Turning Psychoanalytic?," Strupp (1978) commented on some of the converging trends that seemed to be occurring within each of these orientations. Also in the same year, Brown (1978) presented case material reflecting the integration of psychodynamic and behavior therapies, and Ryle (1978) suggested that experimental cognitive psychology might provide a common language for the psychotherapies.

Prochaska (1979), in a textbook describing various approaches to psychotherapy, concluded with a chapter that made the case for ultimately developing a transtheoretical orientation that would encompass what may have been found to be effective across different approaches to psychotherapy. Presenting some interesting parallels between cognitive therapy and psychodynamic therapy, Sarason (1979) suggested that experimental cognitive psychology may provide us with a conceptual system for understanding both orientations. Goldfried (1979) proposed that cognitive-behavior therapy might more usefully be construed as dealing at times with an individual's implicit meaning structures, and that the use of association techniques from experimental cognitive psychology to study such phenomena should be equally acceptable to clinicians and theorists of a psychodynamic orientation. It is interesting to note that the conclusions drawn by Sarason and Goldfried were made independently, and without any apparent knowledge of the very similar conclusion described by Ryle (1978) in the previous year.

Robertson (1979) speculated on some of the reasons for the existence of eclecticism, such as lack of pressures in one's training or professional setting that demand a given viewpoint, the tendency for clinical experience to make a therapist more open to other procedures, a personal tendency to be a nonjoiner, and a therapeutic orientation reaching a point where "the bloom is off the rose." Related to this last point are the results of Mahoney's (1979) survey of leading cognitive and noncognitive behavior therapists. Among the several questions asked of the respondents was: "I feel satisfied with the adequacy of my current understanding of human behavior." Although there were no statistically significant differences between the two groups on this item, the absolute rating was indeed instructive. Using a 7-point scale, Mahoney found that the average rating of satisfaction was less than 2.

The Early 1980s

Making note of past attempts to find commonalities across the psychotherapies, Goldfried (1980a) argued that a fruitful level of abstraction at which such a comparative analysis might take place would be somewhere between the specific technique and the theoretical explanation for the potential effectiveness of that technique. Goldfried maintained that it was at this intermediate level of abstraction — at the level of a clinical strategy — that potential points of overlap could exist. One clinical strategy that may very well cut across orientations entails providing the client with corrective experiences, particularly with regard to fear-related activities. For example, Fenichel (1941), on the topic of fear reduction, noted that:

> when a person is afraid but experiences a situation in which what was feared occurs without any harm resulting, he will not immediately trust the outcome of his new experience; however, the second time he will have a little less fear, the third time still less. (p. 83)

This very same conclusion was reached by Bandura (1969), who observed:

> Extinction of avoidance behavior is achieved by repeated exposure to subjectively threatening stimuli under conditions designed to ensure that neither the avoidance responses nor the anticipated adverse consequences occur. (p. 414)

Relevant to this general theme was an article by Nielsen (1980), who described how certain psychoanalytic concepts were reflected in the practice of gestalt therapy.

In a special issue of *Cognitive Therapy and Research* appearing in 1980, therapists from various orientations responded to the same set of questions about what they believed to be the most effective ingredients associated with therapeutic change (Brady, Davison, Dewald, Egan, Fadiman, Frank, Gill, Hoffman, Kempler, Lazarus, Raimy, Rotter, & Strupp, 1980). Goldfried and Strupp (1980) had a dialogue on the issue of rapprochement at the 1980 AABT Convention, in which they agreed that in the final analysis, any attempt at finding points of commonality must be based on what clinicians do, rather than what they say they do. Marmor and Woods' (1980) edited book *The Interface between the Psychodynamic and Behavioral Therapies* illustrated the theme that no single approach to therapy can deal with all of human functioning. A survey by Larson (1980) indicated that although therapists typically used a single orientation as their primary reference point, 65% acknowledged that their clinical work included contributions made by a number of other therapeutic approaches. Garfield (1980), drawing on different therapeutic orientations, described in *Psychotherapy: An Eclectic Approach* an empirically oriented view of psychotherapy. He viewed the introduction of cognitive variables into behavior therapy as a particularly important advancement, noting:

> Whether or not it really portends a beginning realization of the limitations of a single approach and the possible rapprochement of some of the different emphases in psychotherapy remains to be seen. However, it is a step in this direction, and, therefore, a very welcome development. (p. 290)

Relevant to this point was a convention presentation by Meichenbaum in 1980, in which he acknowledged the importance of considering unconscious as well as conscious processes in the development of our assessment procedures. Ryle (1980), outlined in an unpublished manuscript how cognitive psychology might provide opposing theoretical orientations with a unifying model of various clinical disorders.

A chapter by Landau and Goldfried (1981) described in detail how certain concepts from experimental cognitive psychology (e.g., schema, scripts) could offer the field a most consistent framework within which cognitive, behavioral, and traditional assessment may be fit. Bergin chaired a symposium at the 1981 meetings of the American Psychological Association on "Systematic Eclectic Therapy," in which the participants discussed the growing trends toward convergence among the psychotherapies. In the same year, a small group of clinicians and clinical researchers (Garfield, Goldfried, Horowitz, Imber, Kendall, Strupp, Wachtel, and Wolfe) held an informal, 2-day conference to determine whether clinicians of different orientations could communicate with each other about actual case material. Not attempting to derive any particular product as their goal, the primary objective was to have the opportunity to initiate a dialogue with each other. Also appearing in 1981 was a book by Lazarus that detailed clinical procedures for the practice of multimodal therapy; an article by Rhoads (1981) outlining and illustrating the clinical integration of behavior therapy and psychoanalytic therapy; and a chapter by Gurman (1981) that described how different therapeutic orientations may be fit into a multifaceted empirical approach to marital intervention.

Elaborating on the theme that different therapeutic orientations are needed for a multidimensional intervention approach, Bergin (1982) suggested that nobody attempting to understand the workings of the human body would ever try to invoke a single set of principles. Depending upon which aspect of bodily functioning is of interest, different principles may be required. Thus, principles of fluid mechanics are needed to understand how the heart operates, whereas electrochemical principles are needed for an understanding of neural transmission. A true rapprochement across the psychotherapies is needed, says Bergin, if we are to deal effectively with those complex human problems requiring psychotherapeutic intervention. As a way of illustrating how such rapprochement might be implemented, Mahoney and Wachtel (1982) presented a day-long dialogue and discussion of actual clinical material. In the book *Converging Themes in Psychotherapy*, Goldfried (1982) provided a compendium of articles that dealt with the issue of rapprochement, together with an overview of the current status and future direction in psychotherapy as they relate to the development of a more comprehensive paradigm for intervention.

THE MERITS OF INTEGRATION

We have much to learn from clinicians who are in good contact with clinical reality, be they behavioral, psychodynamic, or experiential in orientation. To the extent that we are able to tap these clinical observations at an appropriate level of abstraction—such as the clinical strategy—we may have at our disposal the starting point of some very fruitful clinical research. As I have suggested elsewhere,

> To the extent that clinicians of varying orientations are able to arrive at a common set of strategies, it is likely that what emerges will consist of robust phenomena, as they have managed to survive the distortions imposed by the therapists' carrying theoretical biases. (Goldfried, 1980a, p. 996)

In essence, such strategies function as clinical heuristics that implicitly guide the efforts of most experienced clinicians during the course of therapy.

A review of the available literature dealing with points of commonality across different therapeutic approaches reveals a number of similarities that have been described at the intermediate level of abstraction (Goldfried & Padawer, 1982). Among these are the initially induced expectations that therapy can be helpful; the client or patient's participation in a therapeutic relationship; the possibility of obtaining an external perspective on one's problems; the encouragement of corrective experiences; and the opportunity to repeatedly test reality. Although the specific techniques that are used to implement each of these strategies may vary from orientation to orientation, the strategies themselves nonetheless represent common threads. And as behavior therapists have started to recognize the important influence of cognitive factors in the origin, maintenance, and change process for various human problems—some of which might not be in the person's immediate awareness—many of the points of similarity are likely to grow between behavior therapy and other orientations.

Although one can enumerate what appear to be common therapeutic strategies cutting across different orientations, the generation of these strategies is based on what therapists "say they do," not what they "actually do." Just as we all have observed that our clients and patients do not always have a totally correct view of their actions, so should we anticipate that we, their therapists, may similarly not be faithful observers of our own therapeutic activities. In the final analysis, what is clearly needed is a more direct empirical test of what similarities actually exist across different orientations. Few therapists strictly adhere to a particular therapeutic orientation in actual practice (cf. Grinker 1976; Hunt, 1971; Klein, Dittman, Parloff, & Gill, 1969; Larson, 1980; Strupp, 1978). In many respects, therapists may very well become "shaped" by their patients or clients during the course of their professional careers, whereby they gradually learn to use those procedures and strategies that they have experienced as being successful. As noted in an earlier chapter, Wachtel (1977) has suggested that there exists a therapeutic "underground," reflecting an unofficial consensus of what experienced clinicians know to be true. Many of these factors are not associated with any particular school, and only rarely does one see them described in the literature.

As a cognitive-behavior therapist, I have become acutely aware of the strengths as well as the limitations associated with behavioral procedures. In reading the psychodynamic, behavioral, and experiential literature, and in my conversations with colleagues who work within these frameworks, it has also become evident that professionals from all orientations are going through a period of self-examination. I believe that we have reached the point in the development of psychotherapy where intellectual and professional honesty demands that each of us, regardless of orientation, acknowledges what we can and cannot successfully do. And in making this acknowledgment, we should also entertain the possibility that our areas of weakness might be complemented by another orientation's area of strength (Goldfried & Padawer, 1982).

BARRIERS TO INTEGRATION

It should be the hope of any serious and dedicated professional that one day the practice of psychotherapy will be guided by a new and more comprehensive paradigm. Am I suggesting that we give up our orientations and pursue this paradigm? Not really. At the same time, I firmly believe that much can be learned to enhance our therapeutic effectiveness by borrowing from other therapeutic orientations.

One possible barrier in the integration of the psychotherapies involves the *language problem*. This is manifested not only by the difficulty in understanding various concepts, but also by an active tuning out when one hears certain buzz words associated with another orientation (e.g., "transference," "warded off conflict and defense," "self-actualization," or "unfinished business."). Although the use of the vernacular may be helpful in facilitating communication, as it was in the special issue of *Cognitive Therapy and Research* (Brady et al., 1980), the field ultimately needs a language system that is tied to a data base. A number of contemporary writers have independently suggested the possibility that a common language may ultimately come from the field of experimental cognitive psychology (Goldfried, 1979; Landau & Goldfried, 1981; Ryle, 1978). Concepts such as "schema," "scripts," and "meta-cognition" have the potential for covering therapeutic phenomena observed by clinicians of varying orientations.

Another barrier to rapprochement has been documented within the sociology of science, which has described the extraordinarily *competitive set of rules* by which the scientific community operates (Merton, 1969). Scientists are encouraged to outdo each other. That this has led to the proliferation of numerous different schools of therapy should come as little surprise, especially in light of the financial benefits that are often associated with following a given orientation. Unless there is some consensus on what constitutes acceptable therapeutic outcome measures, there is little to stop this proliferation. Hopefully, more recent emphases on accountability may help us to arrive at agreed-upon standards for therapeutic effectiveness.

Still another barrier to the integration of the psychotherapies is the fact that the field is comprised of numerous *professional networks*, most of which reflect a particular theoretical outlook. As I have noted elsewhere "without a specific therapeutic orientation, how would we know what journals to subscribe to or which conventions to attend?" (Goldfried, 1980a, p. 996). This is not to say that professional networks are not needed, but rather that the particular kind we now have may not provide us with enough scope to advance the field very much beyond its current point. What I am suggesting is the need for a network of professionals who are interested in taking steps toward the ultimate achievement of some kind of rapprochement and consensus— to determine not only the common elements that may cut across different therapeutic orientations, but also to identify those unique contributions that any particular approach may have to offer. My sense is that there are a growing number of therapists who, while still maintaining their own theoretical identities, are nonetheless willing to explore such potential sources of convergence.

SUMMARY

The hope of finding a way to integrate the various approaches to psychotherapy dates back to the 1930s. This chapter has highlighted the historical trends in this area, which appear to be gaining momentum. Therapists of all orientations are beginning to become more interested in determining common elements that cut across their different frameworks and are starting to acknowledge that characteristics that are unique to other approaches might conceivably complement their own intervention procedures. The documentation of this historical development is concluded by noting some of the barriers that keep the field of psychotherapy from reaching a consensus and ultimately being guided by a new and more comprehensive paradigm.

13

Toward the Delineation of Therapeutic Change Principles

It has been approximately one hundred years since the practice of psychotherapy emerged as a recognized professional activity. Partly as a function of this unofficial anniversary, but more as the result of a growing zeitgeist in the field, the time is ripe for questioning how far we have come and how close we are to achieving a "consensus" (cf. Kuhn, 1970) within the professional community. The thesis developed in this chapter is that psychotherapy is currently in a state of infancy; anyone desiring therapy nowadays needs to decide which of more than 130 different approaches is likely to be most helpful (Parloff, 1976). It will be argued, however, that the time is rapidly approaching when more than ever before, we have the opportunity to advance the field in the direction of greater maturity.

Before developing this thesis, I might note that my original intent was to have the article on which this chapter is based published anonymously, but editorial policy prevented this from happening. The reason for wanting the article to appear anonymously was that all of us interested in the field of psychotherapy seem to have a tendency either to read or to ignore articles and books on the basis of our allegiance with the author's theoretical camp. We have all "taken up sides" and have placed far too much emphasis on *who* is correct, not *what* is correct. I wanted to circumvent this tendency, as I believe the message has relevance to therapists of all orientations.

Much of what is included in this chapter is based on the writings of therapists from psychoanalytic, behavioral, and humanistic orientations. To let them speak for themselves, I have taken the liberty of quoting them liberally. My observation has been that there has been a growing discontent among therapists within each orientation and that the need for rapprochement is becoming ever more appropriate. Although it may be possible to delineate commonalities across all theoretical persuasions, formidable pressures nonetheless exist that oppose such integration. Jerome Frank (1976) has astutely noted such barriers by suggesting that "features which are shared by all therapists have been relatively neglected, since little glory derives from showing that the particular method one has mastered with so much effort may be indistinguishable from other methods in its effects" (p. 74). The goal of this chapter is not to outline these shared features but to suggest what needs to be done to work toward integration.

PSYCHOTHERAPY: APPROACHING A CRISIS

In reviewing the history of various approaches to therapy, it becomes apparent that therapists have typically operated from within a given theoretical framework, often to the point of being completely blind to alternative conceptualizations and potentially effective intervention procedures. Considering the role that schools of therapy have played in the development of the field, Raimy (1976) has observed that these schools "undoubtedly contributed to the enthusiasm and the competitive urge to drive therapists to develop their thinking and their techniques, but also imposed limited horizons which clamped their proponents into rigid molds" (p. 225).

Although examples of this are legion, a few may be offered to illustrate the point: Many of Freud's early attempts to introduce psychoanalytic insights and techniques into the profession were initially ignored, if not explicitly rejected, as they did not fit into the generally accepted theoretical framework at the time. Although procedures for progressive relaxation were originally described by Jacobson in 1929, it took nearly thirty years before the therapeutic potential was recognized. At the time it was introduced, it no doubt appeared superficial and mechanistic and did not "fit" with what was deemed to be necessary for effecting therapeutic change. Breger and McGaugh's (1965) criticism of behavior therapy for its exclusive reliance on classical and operant conditioning principles was initially rejected by behavior therapists, although the cogency of their critique has been acknowledged indirectly by the rapid growth of cognitive-behavior therapy. And though intervention procedures for the treatment of sexual dysfunctions were introduced into the literature in the 1950s (Seamans, 1956; Wolpe, 1958), their professional use was not fully explored until Masters and Johnson (1970) presented their suggestions for the direct treatment of sexual difficulties.

Despite our tendency to be suspicious of new ideas, we do eventually process novel information. During the 1970s, an interesting phenomenon seemed to have emerged. There appeared a slight, but clearly growing trend toward questioning whether or not all the answers may be found within any given school of therapy (e.g., Appelbaum, 1975, 1979; Bergin & Strupp, 1972; Birk & Brinkley-Birk, 1974; Brady, 1968; Burton, 1976; Dewald, 1976; Egan, 1975; Feather & Rhoads, 1972; Ferster, 1974; Frank, 1976; Goldfried & Davison, 1976; Goldstein, 1976; Grinker, 1976; Haley, 1963; Horwitz, 1976; Lazarus, 1977; Lewis, 1972; London, 1972; Marmor, 1971; Martin, 1972; Raimy, 1975, 1976; Ricks, Wandersman, & Poppen, 1976; Segraves & Smith, 1976; Silverman 1974; Wachtel, 1977). We seem to have entered a period of self-examination, with therapists beginning to ask themselves such questions as, Where does our approach fail? What are the limits of our paradigm? Do other approaches have something useful to offer? One gets the impression that therapists started to grow somewhat weary of a strict adherence to their theoretical orientation and became more pragmatic. In surveys of clinical psychologists within the United States (Garfield & Kurtz, 1976; Kelly, Goldberg, Fiske, & Kilkowski, 1978), between 55% and 58% of those professionals contacted indicated that they did not adhere to any single orientation. This eclecticism may have evolved over a period of time or, in some instances, may reflect an integration of different orientations from the outset of their professional training.

Kuhn (1970) has observed that scientific revolutions are typically preceded by a period of "crisis," when well-accepted paradigms simply do not work as well as they did before. Such crises are reflected by the "proliferation of competing articulations, the willingness to try anything, the expression of explicit discontent, the recourse to philosophy and to debate over fundamentals" (p. 91). It appears that just as our clients change their perceptions of the world as a result of corrective experiences, we, their therapists, have become more willing to question our particular paradigm as a result of our own corrective experiences. In some cases this may occur because the therapist is successful with an intervention procedure typically associated with another theoretical orientation. In other instances, such changes appear to be the result of personal therapy with a therapist of a different persuasion.

In light of the historical overview described in Chapter 12, one may argue that the tendency for therapists to look to other approaches for what they may have to offer is nothing new. Moreover, Fiedler (1950) found some years ago that greater similarity was to be found among experienced clinicians of different therapeutic schools than among beginning therapists of varying orientations. Presumably, with increased experience — both clinical and through living itself — more points of commonality emerge. These findings confirm what has frequently been observed among practicing clinicians, namely that there exists a therapeutic underground, which rarely appears in the literature but which nonetheless reflects those informal, if not unspoken, clinical observations on what tends to work (Klein, Dittman, Parloff, & Gill, 1969; Wachtel, 1977). Although this underground may always have been there, we have reached a point when clinicians are acknowledging its existence more openly and are beginning to recognize the contributions from orientations other than their own.

Among psychoanalytically oriented therapists are several instances of this open acknowledgment that other theoretical orientations may have something valuable to contribute. For example, Dewald (1976) has stated that efforts need to be made toward rapprochement, suggesting that "the articulation of conceptual generalizations regarding the therapeutic process in different treatment modalities hopefully might initiate more objective and dispassionate comparison of similarities and differences" (p. 284). As the result of findings from the Menninger Foundation Psychotherapy Research Project, Horwitz (1974, 1976) has concluded that supportive therapeutic procedures, involving no uncovering, were just as effective as insight oriented psychoanalytic therapy. Appelbaum (1979), a former colleague of Horwitz at Menninger, has argued that psychoanalytic therapy can learn much from the intervention procedures used by gestalt therapists. In one of his last papers, Alexander (1963) acknowledged the role of learning theory in the full understanding of the therapeutic process, prophesying the integration of psychoanalytic theory with learning theory. And in a scholarly evaluation of the clinical and theoretical links between psychoanalysis and behavior therapy, Wachtel (1977) has suggested how the two approaches to intervention may effectively be integrated.

Within behavior therapy one sees some similar self-examination and openness to the views of others. As noted earlier, a survey of leading behavior therapists, asking them to rate how satisfied they were with their current understanding of human behavior (Mahoney, 1979), revealed a most noteworthy finding. On the basis of a 7-point rating scale, it was found that the average rating was less than 2! One would certainly never have expected that from reading the behavioral literature. Lazarus (1977), one of the pioneers in the development of behavior therapy, stated his position as follows:

> I am opposed to the advancement of psychoanalysis, to the advancement of Gestalt therapy, to the advancement of existential therapy, to the advancement of behavior therapy, or to the advancement of any delimited school of thought. I would like to see an advancement in psychological knowledge, an advancement in the understanding of human interaction, in the alleviation of suffering, in the know-how of therapeutic intervention. (p. 553)

Davison (1978) and Thoresen (1973) have argued for the possible synthesis of behavioral and humanistic approaches to therapy. And Goldfried and Davison (1976) have appealed to their colleagues to seriously consider a rapprochement by suggesting:

> It is time for behavior therapists to stop regarding themselves as an outgroup and instead to enter into serious and hopefully mutually fruitful dialogues with their nonbehavioral colleagues. Just as we firmly believe that there is much that behavior therapy can say to clinicians of other orientations, we reject the assumption that the slate should be wiped clean and that therapeutic innovations should be — and even can be — completely novel. (p. 15)

Even among those who are primarily Skinnerian in their behavioral emphasis, one saw efforts to draw on other orientations. Thus Ferster (1974) has argued that behavioral and psychodynamic approaches "are complementary rather than exclusive ways to uncover the actual events of psychopathology and the procedures of therapy" (p. 153). Another example can be found in Baer and Stolz's (1978) article in *Behaviorism* on the potential therapeutic effectiveness of *est*.

Among those who are primarily identified with a humanistic orientation, Landsman (1974) emphasized some of the similarities between humanistic and behaviorally oriented intervention approaches, urging his colleagues to recognize the contribution that behavior therapy may have to offer. He suggests:

> If humanists are truly confident that they have much to offer then they ought to welcome what is being offered by the responsible behaviorists—attention to specifics, to details, careful quantification, modesty in claims, demonstrable results. And even beyond this we welcome its challenge, its role as stimulator to make the dreams of humanistic psychology more of the substance of reality, the spur to demonstrate our promises. (p 15)

Egan modified his earlier reviews (Egan, 1970, 1973) of the interpersonal growth process by suggesting that there comes a time when the therapist must assist the client in acting differently in the real world (Egan, 1975). The therapist's goal then becomes "collaborating with the client in working out specific action programs; helping the client to act on his new understanding of himself; exploring with the client a wide variety of means for engaging in constructive behavioral change; giving support and direction to action programs" (Egan, 1975, p. 30). Egan went on to suggest that a useful way of facilitating such direct action is to employ the procedures developed by behavior therapy. In an issue of the *Journal of Humanistic Psychology*, the editor acknowledged Lazarus's (1977) call for a rapprochement across various therapeutic orientations and urged the readers of the journal to be open to such attempts (Greening, 1978). It will be recalled that it was none other than Maslow (1966) who warned us against becoming too firmly entrenched within a given perspective, observing, "If the only tool you have is a hammer, [you tend] to treat everything as if it were a nail" (pp. 15–16).

RAPPROCHEMENT THROUGH COMMON CLINICAL STRATEGIES

In considering how one might approach the task of looking for points of commonality among different orientations, it might be helpful to conceptualize the therapeutic enterprise as involving various levels of abstraction from what is directly observable. At the highest level of abstraction we have the *theoretical framework* to explain how and why change takes place, as well as an accompanying *philosophical stance* on the nature of human functioning. In the search for commonalities, it is unlikely that we can ever hope to reach common ground at either the theoretical or the philosophical level. Indeed, numerous differences can be found at this level within the psychoanalytic, behavioral, and humanistic orientations. At the lowest level of abstraction, we have the therapeutic *techniques* or clinical *procedures* that are actually employed during the intervention process. Although commonalities across approaches may be found in the realm of specific techniques (e.g., role playing, relaxation training), it is unlikely that such comparisons would reveal much more than trivial points of similarity. I would suggest, however, that the possibility of finding meaningful consensus exists at a level of abstraction somewhere between theory and technique which, for want of a better term, we might call *clinical strategies*. Were these strategies to have a clear empirical foundation, it might be more appropriate to call them *principles of change*. In essence, such strategies function as clinical heuristics that implicitly guide our efforts during the course of therapy. For illustrative purposes, I would like to offer as examples two such strategies that may very well be common to all theoretical orientations: (*a*) providing the patient with new, corrective experiences, and (*b*) offering the patient direct feedback.

Therapists of varying orientations have suggested that one of the essential ingredients of change in the clinical setting involves having the client engage in new, corrective experiences (e.g., Grinker, 1976; Marmor, 1976; Prochaska, 1979; Raimy, 1975; Rotter, 1954; Strupp, 1976; Thoresen & Coates, 1978). The role that new experiences play in the clinical change process was initially outlined in Alexander and French's (1946) description of the "corrective emotional experience," which suggested that concurrent life experiences could change patients even without their having had insight into the origins of their problems. Alexander and French emphasized the importance of encouraging their patients to engage in previously avoided actions in order to recognize that their fears and misconceptions about such activities were groundless. They even suggested giving homework assignments to patients so that they would act differently between sessions and facilitate such corrective experiences. In an attempt to justify their more liberal, if not seemingly radical, suggestion, they noted that "Freud himself came to the conclusion that in the treatment of some cases, phobias, for example, a time arrives when the analyst must encourage the patient to engage in those activities he avoided in the past" (Alexander & French, 1946, p. 39). The strategy was noted by Fenichel (1941), who made the following clinical observation:

> When a person is afraid but experiences a situation in which what was feared occurs without any harm resulting, he will not immediately trust the outcome of his new experience; however, the second time he will have a little less fear, the third time still less. (p. 83)

In his analysis of how people change, Wheelis (1973) has suggested, "Personality change follows change in behavior. Since we are what we do, if we want to change what we are we must begin by changing what we do, must undertake a new mode of action" (p. 101). This observation was confirmed by Horwitz's (1974, 1976) report of the Menninger Foundation Psychotherapy Research Project's finding that corrective experiences, provided to patients within the context of supportive therapy, resulted in as much long-lasting therapeutic change as did more traditional psychoanalytic psychotherapy.

In the case of behavior therapy, the same clinical strategy has been employed. Although behavior therapists have tended to place greater emphasis on the observable characteristics of the client's novel behavior patterns, rather than the more subjective experiences, they nonetheless encourage clients to do things in ways they have not tried before. Kanfer and Phillips (1966) refer to this as the "instigation" aspect of behavior therapy, the objective being to encourage the client to respond differently to various life situations. Clients are taught new ways to deal with various situations through role playing and are urged to try out these new behavior patterns as homework assignments (Goldfried & Davison, 1976; Lazarus, 1971; Wolpe, 1973) Although a variety of different behavior therapy procedures have been used in reducing clients' fears and phobias, several behavior therapists have suggested that the overriding clinical strategy involves having clients expose themselves to the feared situation (Agras, 1967; Bandura, 1969; Marks, 1969; Wilson & Davison, 1971). As stated by Bandura (1969), "Extinction of avoidance behavior is achieved by repeated exposure to subjectively threatening stimuli under conditions designed to ensure that neither avoidance responses nor the anticipated adverse consequences occur" (p. 414). Setting aside the behavioral jargon, this conclusion is clearly consistent with Fenichel's clinical observations quoted above.

Among humanistically oriented therapists, one sees a similar strong emphasis on having clients experience change through concerted efforts to behave differently. Thus Schutz (1973) indicated that one of the ground rules of encounter groups involved having clients take risks and attempt to respond differently: "Whatever you are most afraid of is the thing it is most valuable to do" (p. 425). A basic underpinning of gestalt therapy involves the importance of learning through personal experience, going beyond the mere discussion "about" these experiences (Fagan & Shepherd, 1970; Polster & Polster, 1973). One of the ways of furthering this learning is through *directed behavior*, the objective of which is to provide the client with "the opportunity for relevant practice in behaviors he may be avoiding. Through his own discoveries in trying out these behaviors, he will uncover aspects of himself which in their turn will generate further self-discovery" (Polster & Polster, 1973, p. 252).

A second possible clinical strategy that may be common to all therapeutic approaches consists of *direct feedback*, whereby patients are helped to become more aware of what they are doing and not doing, thinking and not thinking, and feeling and not feeling in various situations. One of the first therapists to observe this phenomenon was Reich (1933/1949), who made the following fortuitous observation:

> What is added in character-analysis is merely that we isolate the character trait and confront the patient with it repeatedly until he begins to look at it objectively and to experience it like a painful symptom; thus, the character trait begins to be experienced as a foreign body which the patient wants to get rid of. . . . Surprisingly, the process brings about a change — although only a temporary one — in the personality. (p. 50)

Compare this observation with the more recent serendipitous finding by behavior therapists who, in an attempt to use self-monitoring procedures for assessment purposes, noted that their clients changed merely as a result of observing their own behavior. The typical conclusion reached by behavior therapists is that "when an individual begins paying unusually close attention to one aspect of his behavior, that behavior is likely to change even though no change may be intended or desired" (McFall, 1970, p. 140). The similarity to the phenomenon that Reich unexpectedly uncovered is striking. In gestalt and encounter approaches to therapeutic change, considerable emphasis is placed on offering the client feedback, either from the therapist or from other group members. Bugental (1965) has suggested that providing feedback to the client is an essential component in enhancing personal awareness. And one of the procedural cornerstones of nondirective therapy (Rogers, 1951) has involved the therapist's attempts to reflect back to clients their thoughts and feelings.

There are other clinical strategies that may be common to psychoanalytic, behavioral, and humanistic approaches to therapy, which we will note in the next chapter. I would like to emphasize, however, that my goal here was not to outline all possible commonalities. Instead, it was to illustrate the level of abstraction on which we may need to focus in order to achieve such consensus.

WHERE DO WE GO FROM HERE?

In our attempt to study the effectiveness of our therapeutic procedures, we have expended far too much energy investigating techniques that may not be all that powerful clinically. Far too much time and talent have been spent on the detailed and parametric study of trivial issues. The popularity of comparative therapy research, in which one orientation is pitted against another, similarly has its inherent limitations. To the extent that common elements indeed exist across all approaches to therapy, such a research strategy is likely to undermine any differential effectiveness. Further, if there are inert as well as effective procedures associated with each therapeutic approach studied, such comparative research would not seem to be the most efficient way of uncovering effective intervention procedures. As noted by Luborsky, Singer, and Luborsky (1975), "everybody has won and all must have prizes" (p. 1003).

On the other hand, it would be naïve to conclude that the delineation of commonalities among different approaches to therapy will in itself result in consensus. A likely, although clearly unfortunate, reaction among some might be to conclude that "we're all doing the same thing" and to return complacently to their usual orientation and set of procedures To be an eclectic is to have a marginal professional identity. By contrast, an identification with a school of therapy is likely to result in some very powerful economic, political, and social supports. After all, without a specific therapeutic orientation, how would we know what journals to subscribe to or which conventions to attend? Krasner (1978), in a candid analysis of the past and future in the behaviorism-humanism dialogue, commented on the factors that contribute to the continuation of varying schools of thought, noting:

> In effect, each new slogan and label takes on a full and happy life of its own. I write not as a disinterested historian of this game but rather as a participant-observer with as much guilt (or credit depending on your orientation) as anyone else in the controversy between behaviorism and humanism. (p. 800)

The popularity of a therapy school is often a function of variables having nothing to do with the efficacy of its associated procedures. Among other things, it depends on the charisma, energy level, and longevity of the leader; the number of students trained and where they have been placed; and the spirit of the times. By contrast, there exist certain "timeless truths," consisting of common observations of how people change. These observations date back to early philosophers and are reflected in great works of literature. As suggested throughout this chapter, these observations have also been noted by most experienced and sensitive clinicians. *To the extent that clinicians of varying orientations are able to arrive at a common set of strategies, it is likely that what emerges will consist of robust phenomena, as they have managed to survive the distortions imposed by the therapists' varying theoretical biases.* Although it is clear that a systematic and more objective study of the therapeutic change process is needed to advance our body of knowledge, it would be a grievous error to ignore what has been unsystematically observed by many.

I do not mean to imply that these clinical observations will provide us with all the answers but, rather, that they can offer us an important supplement to, if not a starting point for, other research approaches. Basic research on the origin and maintenance of various psychological disorders is clearly needed as well. I would also like to emphasize that I am not arguing against theory per se, but rather against the very strong temptation to engage in premature speculation. We need to have a clearer consensus on the observable phenomena associated with change before we attempt to theorize about them.

It is presumptuous to expect that any one person will be able to outline a comprehensive model of change. Inasmuch as there exists a gap between theory and practice, any individual from a given orientation can never really be knowledgeable about the therapeutic underground within other orientations. Moreover, the "I-have-the-answers-come-follow-me" message that would accompany any one person's attempt at integration may only serve to put off one's colleagues, or perhaps even end up in the establishment of yet another school of therapy! What is needed instead is a more cooperative effort. Unfortunately this is not always easily achieved. The field of therapy—and certainly other disciplines as well—places too much emphasis on the ownership of ideas, such that we are unwilling to consider the merit of certain notions if they come from those we do not consider to be part of our reference group. Though it would be nice to find cooperative efforts naturally occurring among scientists, it is perhaps more realistic to expect their behavior to reflect the competitiveness inherent in our society at large. Noting how the scientist's early desire to forward a common goal often falls by the wayside, David and Brannon (1976) have observed that "many students are originally attracted to science by [the] image of noncompetitive sharing, only to find a few years later that they are in a system not unlike the competitive world of business they once disdained" (p. 143)

It is no easy task to get us to set aside our well-established, if not time-honored, practice of setting one approach against another and, instead, to work toward a rapprochement. What may be needed to get us to mobilize our cooperative efforts is *an attack from outside the system itself.* This clearly was the case during World War II, when scientists found themselves working cooperatively toward common goals. In the case of psychotherapy, there is a strong possibility that the attack from outside may come from questions associated with third-party payments. The pressure from governmental agencies and insurance companies—as well as the growing consumer movement—to have us demonstrate the efficacy of our intervention procedures may very well serve as the necessary impetus for the cooperative effort the field so sorely needs. In a stimulating and challenging account of policymakers' growing interest in the empirical foundations of psychotherapy, Parloff (1979) pointed out that

> members of our new audience are raising very pragmatic, prosaic, yet profound questions regarding the efficacy of the wide range of psycho-

social interventions currently offered to the public. Clinicians and government officials are experiencing mounting pressures from such not easily disregarded sources as the courts, insurance companies, and national health insurance planners. Third-party payers—ultimately the public—are demanding crisp and informative answers to questions regarding the quality, quantity, durability, safety, and efficiency of psychosocial treatments provided to an ever-widening range of consumers and potential consumers. (p. 297)

My fantasy is that we have a working conference directed toward the goal of developing the field of therapy, not toward the advancement of any given school of thought or of any one individual's career. Parenthetically, it might be noted that Rogers (1963) called for a similar dialogue and search for commonalities some years ago, but the zeitgeist may not have been as hospitable at that time. In the hypothetical conference I am suggesting, the participants would include practicing clinicians of varying theoretical persuasions who would be willing to sit down and outline intervention strategies. Such a dialogue would ultimately need to include the direct observation of what actually occurs during the therapeutic process. These clinicians would not be asked to give up their own particular orientation, but to take steps to work toward some consensus. In breaking set and looking for commonalities, we might even find ourselves more willing to acknowledge the unique contributions that other orientations have to offer. Also present at this conference would be individuals who have been involved in therapy research. Their task would be to guide the discussion in such a way that the strategies outlined can be operationalized and put to empirical test.

It is my hope that the resulting research would address itself to the parametric considerations associated with each potentially robust clinical strategy, as it is not likely that a given strategy would apply to all problems and under all circumstances. This point has been made time and again by therapists of varying persuasions: "*What* treatment, by *whom*, is most effective for *this* individual with *that* specific problem, and under *which* set of circumstances?" (Paul, 1967, p. 111); "The challenging question is not which technique is better than all others, but under what circumstances and for what conditions is the particular technique or particular kind of therapist more suitable than another" (Marmor, 1976, p. 8); and "What kinds of changes are affected by what kinds of techniques applied to what kinds of patients by what kinds of therapists under what kinds of conditions?" (Parloff, 1979, p. 303). Thus, if new, corrective experiences were seen as a common strategy, one would need to investigate the most effective tactic or technique for providing such experiences (e.g., individually, in groups, in imagination, via role playing, face to face), the number and nature of such experiences, the optimal level of emotional arousal needed for change to occur, and the extent to which the particular method of implementing the strategy interacts with other client and therapist variables. On the topic of direct feedback, one might want to study the source of such feedback (e.g., therapist, self, peer, significant other) and how these specific procedures interact with other relevant variables.

Whatever merits there may be to what I have suggested, one needs to be realistic and, again, to recognize that this is by no means an easy path to pursue. Just as patients often find it difficult to develop a new view of the world, so it is difficult for us to relinquish our theoretical paradigms. Kuhn (1970) has documented the reluctance of scientists to undergo a shift in paradigm, noting,

> The source of resistance is the assurance that the older paradigm will ultimately solve all its problems, that nature can be shoved into the box the paradigm provides. Inevitably, at times of revolution, that assurance seems stubborn and pigheaded as indeed it sometimes becomes. (pp. 151-152)

Happily, Kuhn goes on to observe,

> Though some scientists, particularly the older and more experienced ones, may resist indefinitely, most of them can be reached in one way or another. Conversions will occur a few at a time until, after the last holdouts have died, the whole profession will again be practicing under a single, but now different paradigm. (p. 152)

Clearly, we need to rewrite our textbooks on psychotherapy. In picking up the textbook of the future, we should see in the table of contents *not* a listing of School A, School B, and so on — perhaps ending with the author's attempt at integration — but an outline of the various agreed-upon intervention principles, a specification of varying techniques for implementing each principle, and an indication of the relative effectiveness of each of these techniques together with their interaction with varying presenting problems and individual differences among clients and therapists. I sense that the time is rapidly approaching when serious, if not painstaking, work on gathering the necessary information for such a text can begin.

SUMMARY

During the 1970s, psychoanalytic, behavioral, and humanistically oriented clinicians raised serious questions about the limits of their respective approaches and started to become more open to contributions from other paradigms. This chapter has documented this phenomenon, which resembles a Kuhnian-type crisis. It has also noted some of the political, economic, and social forces apt to affect our likelihood of ever reaching a consensus within the field, and presented an approach to the delineation and study of common clinical strategies across various orientations.

14

Key Issues in Psychotherapy Integration

I first experienced the paradigm strain of therapeutic orientations in a very personal way during the late 1970s, while I was demonstrating cognitive-behavior therapy to graduate students behind a one-way mirror. As I was working with a particular client, I found myself continually confronted with the same dilemma, namely, should I do what my clinical sense suggested or should I respond as a behavior therapist was *supposed* to respond? My internal dialogue went something as follows:

> This client really needs to get in touch with her feelings, and that's what we should probably be working on at this point. But wait a minute. We can't do that. That would no longer be "behavior therapy," and this is supposed to be a behavior therapy demonstration. For me to shift my approach at this point would only confuse the students. On the other hand, if I were *really* working with this woman clinically, that's the direction I would take. Why do I have this strange feeling that it would be "cheating" if I did something that wasn't officially behavior therapy?

To be sure, most practicing clinicians rarely have the opportunity to demonstrate a specific approach, and consequently may not have experienced this particular conflict. Nonetheless, I would suspect that most therapists have had numerous occasions to question the adequacy of their approach with a particular case, and have struggled with the issue of working with patients in ways that depart from their identified orientation. And if they have taken the time to step back and examine the therapeutic enterprise as a whole, they may have reached the conclusion that a complete understanding of the intricacies of human functioning, and the existence of comprehensive guidelines for changing such functioning, go beyond the scope of any one orientation. The awareness of these limitations, and the dissatisfaction with existing schools, have given rise to the growing interest in rapprochement among the psychotherapies.

There exists a surprisingly extensive literature that deals directly with rapprochement and therapeutic integration. A bibliography compiled in 1984 (Goldfried & Wachtel, 1984) yielded a total of 125 articles, 27 chapters, and 36 books specifically devoted to the topic. One year later, an additional 11 books on the topic were found to have been, or were in the process of being published (Goldfried & Wachtel 1985). And yet, this issue has consisted more of a latent theme than an explicit area of interest. This became evident in the process of working on the bibliography, particularly in attempting to conduct a computer search of the *Psychological Abstracts*. The use of such search terms as "rapprochement," "eclecticism," and "psychotherapy integration" yielded only a handful of references. Clearly, the references existed; it was just that no one had deemed it an important enough area to index.

This chapter begins with a description of what appears to be common elements among, as well as unique contributions from the psychodynamic, behavioral, and experiential orientations. Some of the potential barriers that have traditionally prevented work on integration are discussed, including the different language systems used from one orientation to another, and the existence of professional networks that have been built around specific schools of thought. Finally, the formation of the Society for the Exploration of Psychotherapy Integration (SEPI) is described, the purpose of which is to encourage future clinical and research efforts in this area.

INTEGRATION: COMMONALITIES AND COMPLEMENTARITIES

It is profitable to consider the integration of the psychotherapies from two general vantage points. One is to look for points of commonality that characterize virtually all approaches to therapy. As suggested in Chapter 13, the general assumption here is that any points of commonality that exist among systems having very different starting points may be able to provide us with potentially "robust phenomena," as they have managed to emerge despite the theoretical biases of the different orientations. The second general approach is based on the assumption that different therapy orientations have tended to focus more on certain aspects of human functioning and the change process more than have others, and that any comprehensive system of intervention might fruitfully draw on the complementary nature of these different emphases.

Commonalities

As indicated in the historical review of integration outlined in Chapter 12, the search for common ingredients in psychotherapy dates back to the 1930s. Despite these early efforts, the field has not yet been able to achieve any consensus on this issue. Also noted in an earlier chapter, one reason for this lack of consensus was offered by Frank (1976), who suggested that "features which are shared by all therapists have been relatively neglected . . . (because) little glory derives from showing that the particular method one has mastered with so much effort may be indistinguishable from other methods in its effects" (p. 74).

Quite apart from such personal obstacles — as well as social, political, and economic barriers, some of which we shall return to later in the chapter — the difficulty in arriving at a common set of ingredients among the therapies seems to have been a result of the unit that has been selected in comparing the different approaches. For example, I have argued that the philosophical and theoretical underpinnings among the therapies are so basically different that consensus is impossible. If one were to look for agreement at this level of abstraction, however, the search would be sure to be futile. Making comparisons at the lowest level of abstraction, on the other hand, while it might yield topographical similarities (e.g., reflection of feeling, asking open-ended questions), is likely to result in trivial, nonfunctional points of overlap. As suggested in Chapter 13, meaningful and attainable common ingredients are more likely to be found at a level of abstraction somewhere *between* theory on the one hand, and observable techniques on the other. In this middle level of abstraction, we are more likely to find general clinical strategies or principles that are reflected within all approaches to intervention. The specific methods of implementing these strategies or principles are likely to vary from one orientation to another, as would the theoretical explanations that are offered for the potential effectiveness of the clinical methods. Nonetheless, the middle level principles would be the same.

Although the field of psychotherapy has not yet reached any consensus on common ingredients, a number of writers have addressed themselves to this issue over the years. In a review of this literature, Goldfried and Padawer (1982) have come up with a list of similarities that appear to exist at the intermediate level of abstraction. These include:

The culturally induced expectation that therapy can be helpful.
Based primarily on the work of Frank (1961), who has documented how therapy—as well as other forms of "healing" and personal influence—carries with it a placebo effect, a number of writers have similarly concluded that all interventions serve to enhance an individual's expectations for improvement. By fostering such hope, therapy is able to restore one's sense of morale that may have been lacking prior to therapy.

The participation in a therapeutic relationship.
By becoming involved in a relationship with an attentive, understanding, and nurturing therapist, clients are able to experience an interaction that is likely to be very unique in their life. This experience, in itself, is believed by many to have a beneficial or "therapeutic" effect.

The possibility of obtaining an external perspective on oneself and world.
By providing patients with various forms of feedback—on their thinking, feelings, actions, and the effects that these have on their lives—therapists provide a more objective perspective on what previously might have consisted of a subjective, distorted, and self-defeating outlook. As is the case with other more general principles of change, the specific methods of providing such feedback can take different forms, such as clarification, reflection, interpretation, self-observation or bibliotherapy.

The encouragement of corrective experiences.
One of the crucial aspects of therapeutic change involves having clients be-

have in ways they may have avoided in the past, so as to have the opportunity to experience the absence of negative consequences they may have heretofore feared. Although there may be differences of opinion as to whether or not these critical experiences should take place between sessions or within the session itself, there seems to be agreement that novel experiences are central to the change process.

The opportunity to repeatedly test reality.   This is actually a combination of the two previously mentioned principles—external perspective and corrective experiences—whereby patients continually observe how their distorted view of themselves and others are manifested in their daily life experiences, and at the same time make repeated efforts to behave differently so as to correct these distortions and their accompanying emotions and behavior patterns.

It should be emphasized that these principles are based on what therapists believe to be the active ingredients in psychotherapy. For the most part, it reflects what they say they do, and not independent observations of what they actually do that works. In essence, then, it provides us with a starting point for a step that has yet to be taken, namely the empirical investigation of common principles of change.

Complementarities

It would be unfortunate if our search for common principles of change led us to conclude that we should continue to do what we have always done. The existence of common principles does not necessarily imply that all methods of implementing these principles are interchangeable. Whether one method of providing feedback is generally more effective than another—in general or under certain instances—is clearly a question that can only be answered through research. Thus, the possibility exists that the clinical methods derived from one school of therapy might be a more effective way of implementing a given principle than a method typically used by another orientation. Rather than looking at this line of research as a "test" of one orientation against another, however, it might be more profitable to view it as the parametric study of the means by which a particular principle may be effectively implemented.

There is still another way that different orientations may have something unique to offer in the ultimate development of a comprehensive approach to intervention. As noted in an earlier chapter, Bergin (1982) has pointed out that a thorough understanding of the working of the human body requires more than a single set of principles. Thus, the principles of fluid mechanics needed to explain the way the heart pumps blood through the body are radically different from the electrochemical principles required to understand how impulses are transmitted through neurons. By virtue of their differential emphasis on different aspects of human functioning, psychodynamic, behavioral, and experiential orientations to intervention may each provide a unique contribution.

Psychotherapy, as practiced from within a psychodynamic orientation, has placed a very strong emphasis on understanding the idiosyncratic meaning that individuals give to various life situations, as well as the maladaptive patterns of interpersonal relations that accompany such perceptions. They have called our attention to the role the therapeutic relationship may play in providing us with a sample of the patient's problems, and have alerted us to the ways that the therapist's personal reactions may either help or hinder us in bringing about change.

Behavior therapy has been unique in its development of detailed methods for encouraging corrective experiences, construing a client's problems in terms of variables that can be worked with in a graduated, systematic fashion. There has also been an emphasis on the importance of environmental influences in a person's life. Further, the clear specification of therapeutic guidelines has contributed greatly to the field's development of treatment manuals, important for both therapy research and clinical training. Finally, behavior therapy has highlighted the importance of applying basic research findings to the clinical setting, and has developed research methods for studying the effectiveness of our therapeutic interventions.

Beginning with the pioneering work of Carl Rogers, experiential approaches to therapy have emphasized the importance of the therapist establishing a caring and understanding relationship with the client. They have underscored the need to help clients become better aware of their emotional states, often with the aid of ingenious exercises. The experiential therapies have had much to say about the covert patterns of interaction that exist within intimate relationships, and have contributed to a better understanding of communication patterns required for marital and family interventions.

OVERCOMING BARRIERS TO INTEGRATION

To discuss the merits of rapprochement among the psychotherapies without considering the forces that prevent this from occurring is to deny a very formidable reality. Two of these barriers involve the varying language systems used by different orientations, and the absence of a professional network that can support integrative efforts.

Language Systems

A major obstacle that has existed in our attempts at rapprochement among the therapies has been the different language systems used within each orientation. The fact that we speak in our own unique jargon prevents us from sharing common or complementary clinical observations, experiences, and empirical findings. But there is more than a simple lack of understanding that is at issue here. Quite often, there is an active avoidance, and indeed downright condemnation of concepts used by orientations other than our own. These negative reactions can be set off—depending on your own particular orientation—by terms such as "contingencies," "therapeutic manipulation," and "maintaining variables"; or, "warded off content and defense," "object loss," and "dynamic focus"; or, "unfinished business," "genuineness," and "becoming."

Unless the different approaches to therapy can find a common language with which to dialogue, it is unlikely that we can ever hope to attain any integration. One possibility is to make use of the language that is known by all therapists, namely the vernacular. Long before we were inculcated in the use of our own particular set of jargon, we all spoke about human functioning in non-technical terms. The problem here, however, is that many of the phenomena we see clinically may not be easily construed in the vernacular. Most of us have become so accustomed to our own theoretical language that we find it difficult to think, let alone talk about certain clinical problems in any other way. Nonetheless, there are occasions when it *is* possible to make this translation, at times making it evident that different approaches may really be saying much the same thing. Take, for example, the quotes reported in Chapter 13 by a behavior therapist and psychodynamic therapist about the importance of corrective experiences. In referring to fearful behavior, Bandura (1969) said the following:

Extinction of avoidance behavior is achieved by repeated exposure to subjectively threatening stimuli under conditions designed to ensure that neither avoidance responses nor the anticipated adverse consequences occur. (p. 414)

Compare that conceptualization of the change process to the statement made by Fenichel (1941) who, at the time, was writing in the vernacular:

When a person is afraid but experiences a situation in which what was feared occurs without any harm resulting, he will not immediately trust the outcome of his new experience; however, the second time he will have a little less fear, the third time still less. (p. 83)

To be sure, Bandura and Fenichel may not have used the same therapeutic procedures to bring about such change. Nonetheless, it appears as if they are referring to the same principle of change, namely corrective experiences.

It is helpful to address the issue of a common language from a functional vantage point, considering the *use or uses* to which such a language may be put. At a National Institute of Mental Health (NIMH) workshop on research in psychotherapy integration (Wolfe & Goldfried, 1988), it was pointed out that the language of psychotherapy may be used in four different ways; 1) to facilitate communication within a given orientation; 2) to retrieve basic research findings; 3) to dialogue across orientations; and 4) to conduct comparative psychotherapy process research.

Communicating within a given orientation.   In order to communicate with "like-minded" colleagues, we typically make use of the jargon associated with our own particular orientation. To the extent that we are comfortable in the use of our theoretical constructs, we at times may not even be aware that we are speaking in a unique language system. By the use of terms to refer to complex clinical events and change processes, we have at our disposal an efficient means for communicating with others of a comparable orientation and keeping abreast of the literature. Unfortunately, this body of information is rarely shared with colleagues of a different orientation. Indeed, the exclusionary characteristic of our theoretically based language systems is what has led to the controversy of seeking out a common language.

Retrieving basic research findings. Ryle's (1987) discussion of cognitive psychology as a common language is based on the assumption that there is no discontinuity between human behavior as it occurs within the laboratory and within the clinic setting. As a result, there is the clear implication that research findings in basic psychology may be used to understand the human change process as it occurs within a therapeutic setting. One may argue, then, that it would be most fruitful to translate key constructs from various schools of therapy into a language system that would allow us to retrieve basic research findings from the psychological literature and apply it to the therapeutic situation.

When Ryle discusses cognitive variables, however, he appears to be using the vernacular more than experimental cognitive psychology. Among the various concepts in cognitive psychology that would seem to be relevant to psychotherapy are "schemas," "scripts," and "metacognition." For example, Wachtel (1981) has applied the schema concept to conceptualize the phenomenon of transference. The schemas that we develop in our interaction with other people, suggests Wachtel, tend to remain unaltered because of the absence of direct and unambiguous feedback that is needed to correct any inaccurate schemas. Consequently, misperceptions that clients have of their therapists in psychoanalytic therapy, Wachtel goes on to say, need to be updated by means of clear therapeutic feedback.

A particular type of schema that is most appropriate and suitable for understanding the concept of transference is that of the "personal script" (Schank & Abelson, 1977). Like other scripts, personal scripts involve various components, including the entry condition (when a script seems appropriate), role expectations for the actor and other people involved, as well as specified sets of actions. A script is said to be "personal" when it appears to be determined more by the individual him- or herself, as opposed to the socially acceptable requirements of the situation. The script for interacting with a therapist contains a number of attributes that may overlap with attributes an individual has in his or her script for interacting with a parent (e.g. dealing with an authority figure, asking for assistance). Because of these overlapping attributes, patients may confuse the two scripts.

Another area where scriptal analysis may be useful clinically is in understanding difficulties some individuals have in intimate relationships with a spouse. Here, too, there can be some confusion with scripts learned earlier in life—by observing or interacting with one's parents—as there may exist overlapping attributes associated with scripts for intimate interactions with significant others. The therapeutic task of dealing with the transference or helping individuals improve their intimate relationships essentially involves having patients more clearly define the appropriate script for such interactions in their current life situation. Drawing upon the available research findings about scripts may help us to enhance our therapeutic interventions. I might also add that this is a two-way street, in that our clinical observations of the phenomena that are being researched may conceivably provide our experimental colleagues with important hypotheses for future research.

Dialoguing across orientations.   In the spirit of providing a common language that would be comprehensive enough to deal with a wide array of clinical phenomena, we may make use of the vernacular. In order to translate our various theoretical constructs into the vernacular, however, we would need to engage in a certain amount of conceptual clarification, so that the important concepts associated with our orientation can be made clear to those outside of our frame of reference. Although not an end in itself, the use of the vernacular may help us to clarify much of the confusion and misunderstanding we have developed about other forms of therapy.

It is interesting to note that in the history of medicine, the vernacular was first used by a controversial 16th century physician called Paracelsus (Debus, 1966). He argued that the medical literature at the time was couched in excessive theoretical speculation, which he believed served as an obstacle to progress. Credited with setting forth the foundation for the contemporary experimental approach to the field of medicine, Paracelsus maintained that an unambiguous description of medical phenomena would provide a stronger basis for effective medical practices.

Conducting comparative process research.   Although the vernacular may provide us with a comprehensive second language for communicating with colleagues having orientations different from our own, still another language is needed if we are to engage in actual research on the process of therapeutic change. In addition to translating our concepts into the vernacular, an associated research language is needed. What this refers to is an attempt to operationalize the vernacular so as to allow for a common metric with which to conduct process research. The basic difference between this language system and the vernacular used to dialogue across orientations has to do with its codability within a research context. Thus, in carrying out research on the concept of transference, we might refer to a link made between the patient's perception of a parent and the therapist, which could be reliably coded by independent raters. To the extent that such an operationally defined and codable language system is stated in ordinary language, there is a greater likelihood that research findings using such a methodology could be readily understood by therapists of varying orientations.

Professional Networks

It has been well documented within the sociology of science that scientific fields operate according to a highly competitive set of rules, in which scientists are encouraged to outdo each other (Merton, 1969). Prizes are won for discovering something new, not for confirming someone else's findings. In the natural sciences, where it is easier to obtain some sort of consensus among researchers on how a given phenomenon might be measured, such competition is able to yield agreed-upon discoveries. In the field of psychotherapy, where it is harder to define positive therapeutic outcome, competition among workers in the field is more likely to result in the proliferation of different schools of thought. And because the criterion for therapeutic "success" is so illusive, different schools of therapy are able to stay alive by virtue of the leaders' ability to encourage a following. In addition to the personal involvement associated with one's particular orientation, there are often powerful economic factors—in the form of training institutes and referral networks—that serve to maintain the status quo.

Although our available therapeutic orientations have helped us to create some sense of order out of the complex and often confusing nature of human behavior and the process of change, they have, at the same time, limited our perspective. The same holds true for many of our professional organizations, especially those that are dedicated to the furtherance of a particular school of thought.

In 1979, Hans Strupp and I recognized the field's need for a more comprehensive reference group, one that would be more sympathetic to rapprochement among the therapies. We compiled a list of professionals who we thought might be interested in efforts toward therapeutic integration — not only across theoretical orientations, but also between clinical and research work — and sent them the following letter:

> We are writing this letter to a group of individuals interested in the advancement of psychotherapy, in the hope of establishing an informal network of researchers and clinicians who would like to see a better "working alliance" between research in and the practice of psychotherapy. Although varying theoretical orientations have clearly been useful in helping us to develop a wide variety of therapeutic procedures, we see a need to make greater use of what actually goes on clinically as a way of generating fruitful research hypotheses. Without such close links between clinician and researcher, we face the danger of our theory and research becoming too far removed from the clinical foundations of our generalizations.
>
> Just as we believe that neither the clinician nor the researcher, working alone, can be successful in advancing the field, so do we maintain that no one theoretical orientation can provide us with all the answers. We need to take a close look at the points of commonality that cut across different orientations, as well as the unique contributions that each has to offer. With growing demands for therapists to be accountable for the efficacy of their procedures, the time may be increasingly ripe for clinicians and researchers of various theoretical persuasions to begin to mobilize collaborative efforts.
>
> At this point in time, we are writing to find out whether you would be interested in having your name included on an informal mailing list, which would be distributed to others sympathetic to the general philosophy we have described above. We believe that such a list would enable individuals to more readily identify others sharing this general viewpoint, and could be used to exchange reprints on topics of mutual interest and for purposes of generating symposia, workshops, or conferences.

The response to this inquiry was quite favorable, allowing us to compile and distribute a list of professionals interested in the integration of the psychotherapies. Having reached this point, the question became one of what to do with this network. This question was discussed at great length by Paul Wachtel and myself during luncheon meetings we had over a period of months. I think that the symbolic commitment to actually do something with this informal network came when Wachtel and I realized that we needed to meet for dinner! Taking the list that we already had, and expanding it on the basis of the correspondence we each had with other professionals over the years on the topic of therapy integration, we mailed out a questionnaire in the fall of 1982. A total of 162 individuals completed the questionnaire, indicating that they continued to be interested in rapprochement, and offering their viewpoints on the possible future of this informal network.

The questionnaire asked for their opinions about starting a journal "devoted to theoretical, clinical, and research issues associated with expanding the boundaries of therapeutic schools." Of those responding, 65 percent indicated "yes," with the remaining 35 percent not thinking it was a good idea. Those who were in favor of establishing a journal argued that it might help to combat the fragmentation that characterized the field, encourage the publication of more articles dealing with therapeutic integration, and provide a means by which interested therapists could identify with such efforts. Those having reservations pointed out that there probably was little in the way of high-quality work that could fill the journal, that publishing in existing journals would be more likely to reach a wider audience, and—at least at that point in time—might paradoxically serve to add to, rather than combat fragmentation.

Another question included in the questionnaire was whether or not we should form an organization. To this question, 72 percent thought it was a good idea, and 28 percent said "no" or had serious reservations. As in the response to the inquiry about starting a journal, the numbers alone did not fully reflect the sentiments of the group. Those answering "yes" showed a remarkable degree of enthusiasm about forming an organization, to the point of indicating that they would be willing to volunteer their time to work on its behalf. Some of the responses included:

> "Such an organization would serve as a safe harbor for persons who are often on the cutting edge of thinking in the field and who feel (and often are) alienated by their more conventional colleagues."

"I'm in favor of an organization for the same reason I'm in favor of a journal. It would help to reassure people who are interested in rapprochement that they're not alone and provide them with an opportunity for communication with other like-minded individuals."

"I'm delighted that you are taking this initiative. It is long overdue. We need institutional support of this type to combat the fragmentation of the psychotherapeutic endeavor in dogmatic little camps."

Those who indicated that they were opposed to forming an organization were concerned that it might undermine the kind of informal interaction that was needed in this area, and that the group might end up becoming still another "school" of therapy. Every attempt was made to keep these reservations in mind during our efforts to form an organization, as will be described below.

In a later discussion of the results of the questionnaire, Goldfried and Wachtel (1983) made the following informal observation:

> Two final notes about the questionnaire that convey, we think, why now is the time for such a newsletter and such an organization. Firstly, we have never seen so many exclamation points in response to a questionnaire. We will not be a society of the bland leading the bland; there are strong feelings about many of the issues, both therapeutic and organizational. Secondly, we offer a comment made in Allen Bergin's questionnaire, which captures some of our own feelings about how far we have come in a relatively short time. "I am totally amazed," he said, "to see some of the names on your list." Yes, people one would never have expected to go outside their own reference group have indicated at least some interest in this endeavor. (p. 3)

Wachtel and I left that memorable dinner meeting feeling excited about the prospects and at the same time somewhat frightened by the implications of what we were contemplating. In addition, we felt very much *overwhelmed* by all that needed to be done. Consequently, we contacted four other individuals—Lee Birk, Jeanne Phillips, George Stricker, and Barry Wolfe—and formed an organizing committee.

The organizing committee met for the first time in New York City on June 15, 1983, during which time we discussed the results of the questionnaire. It was immediately apparent to all six of us that the time was ripe to do something with this rapidly growing informal network. Although approximately two thirds of the respondents thought we should start a journal, we ultimately went along with those who thought the time was not yet ripe. This decision was based on the observation that the responses of those opposing the establishing of a journal seemed more passionate, and that the comments of many of those in favor were ambivalent, often including concerns about the timing of such a journal. Instead, the establishment of a newsletter was endorsed by all as the most appropriate way of communicating with those on the network list.

We also discussed the advisability of creating an organization, especially in light of some of the reservations expressed in the questionnaire regarding formalizing something that might best be dealt with informally. In the final analysis, we concluded that *without* the existence of some sort of organization, it would be difficult to maintain any sense of continuity. As later noted by Goldfried and Wachtel (1983), "It was concluded that we needed to achieve a delicate balance: a formal organization that would facilitate informal contacts among the members" (p. 3). Hence, the Society for the Exploration of Psychotherapy Integration — SEPI — was formed.

The network list from which SEPI was born reflected diverse orientations and interests. There were professionals who clearly identified themselves with a particular theoretical framework but openly acknowledged that other schools had something to offer; individuals who were interested in finding commonalities among the therapies; those who wanted to find a way to integrate existing approaches; those who hoped to eventually develop a totally new approach based on research findings; and professionals who had gradually drifted away from their original orientation and were interested in developing clearer guidelines that were more consistent with their clinical experience. A common thread that ran through this diversity was a respect for research evidence and an openness to anything that could be demonstrated to be clinically effective. Goldfried and Wachtel described SEPI as an umbrella organization that was designed to serve the following purposes:

> To begin with, it will function as a reference group for those professionals interested in working toward the development of an approach to psychotherapy that is not necessarily associated with a single theoretical orientation. There are many in the field who find it difficult to align themselves with any particular persuasion, and consequently would

probably welcome such a group with which they can identify. A second function of the society is educational, directed toward those practitioners who may be looking for clearer clinical guidelines, not tied to a specific orientation, within which they might operate. To fulfill this need, conferences, workshops, and reading materials will be made available to the membership. A third function of the society will be to serve those members who might be interested in becoming involved in ongoing collaborative research on the process of psychotherapy. (Goldfried & Wachtel, 1983, p. 4)

Just as the membership of SEPI reflects a wide array of varying orientations, so did the original Advisory Board represent different therapeutic viewpoints and professional orientations. We were truly fortunate to have obtained the support of a distinguished group of individuals, consisting of Aaron T. Beck, Allen E. Bergin, Gerald C. Davison, Irene Elkin, Herbert Fensterheim, Jerome D. Frank, Sol L. Garfield, Merton M. Gill, Alan S. Gurman, Marjorie H. Klein, Harold I. Lief, Perry London, Michael J. Mahoney, Judd Marmor, Donald H. Meichenbaum, Martin T. Orne, Morris B. Parloff, Jeanne S. Phillips, Douglas H. Powell, John M. Rhoads, Laura N. Rice, David A. Shapiro, Hans H. Strupp, Robert S. Wallerstein, and Sherwyn Woods. The membership of SEPI continues to grow, and provides a critical mass of professionals interested in devoting their energies in working toward the integration of the psychotherapies.

SUMMARY

This chapter has considered some of the clinical strategies common to all therapeutic orientations, as well as the unique contributions that the psychodynamic, behavioral and experiential traditions have brought to the therapeutic enterprise. The problem of the different language systems associated with different orientations was also discussed, together with possible solutions. Also described is the origin of the Society for the Exploration of Psychotherapy Integration, the goal of which is to encourage further integrative clinical and research efforts.

15

The Future of Psychotherapy Integration

Predicting the future is a risky business, and trying to anticipate future directions in psychotherapy is certainly no exception. After painstaking interviews and extensive correspondence with leading psychotherapy researchers, Bergin and Strupp (1972) concluded that collaborative research on psychotherapy seemed neither feasible nor warranted. A decade later, NIMH launched its collaborative research program for the treatment of depression (Elkin, Parloff, Hadley & Autry, 1985).

One of the reasons why such predictions are difficult to make is that the sources of change in science are often unexpected and uncontrollable. Thus, although we like to think that advances in psychotherapy are based on empirical research, clinical observations and theoretical contributions emerging from within the field, sociologists have carefully documented how scientific disciplines are strongly influenced by external economic, political, or military factors (Cole & Cole, 1973; Merton, 1938/70). For example, the prospect of adopting national health insurance in the United States in the 1970s provided a renewed impetus within psychotherapeutic circles to demonstrate the effectiveness of our intervention procedures. Although the potential adoption of such an insurance program became less of a concern in the 1980s, the "attack from outside the system" was replaced by the possibility that biological psychiatry might deal as effectively, or perhaps even more effectively than, our existing psychosocial interventions.

In summary, any attempt to predict the future of psychotherapy is undermined by forces about which we can neither know nor control.

Having made this disclaimer, we will attempt to address the questions: (1) where psychotherapy is heading, (2) what the future of integrative approaches might be, and (3) what the integration movement might contribute to psychotherapy.

WHERE IS PSYCHOTHERAPY HEADING IN THE FUTURE?

Over the last two decades, there has been an overwhelming proliferation of different approaches to therapy, reaching the point where over 400 different systems have been tallied (Kazdin, 1986b). Although typically falling within the general categories of psychodynamic, behavioral, experiential, and systemic approaches, there seems to have existed a free market spirit that has characterized the field, where a wide array of diverse therapeutic options were viewed as being healthy and good. However, as suggested by Goldfried and Padawer (1982), "there nonetheless comes a time when one needs to question where fruitful diversity ends and where chaos begins" (p. 3). Our sense is that a growing number of therapists are beginning to raise this very question.

Consolidation and Rapprochement of Clinical Orientations

Many of the new therapies proposed in the 1970s appear to have been passing fads, originally gaining popularity because of the open spirit of the times and the charismatic nature of the leader, rather than the potential efficacy of the methods themselves. Many of these methods have fallen by the wayside, and there appears to be of a return by therapists to more "mainstream" orientations.

With this narrowing of the bewildering array of therapeutic orientations, we may anticipate a greater consolidation of the more traditional therapeutic orientations, as well as a stronger concern for rapprochement across these major approaches. Indeed, it would not be surprising if we saw future generations of therapists choosing to be trained in one particular traditional orientation, while at the same time showing a greater openness toward the theoretical, clinical, and empirical contributions of other approaches.

In large part due to the influential writings of such authors as

Frank (1973), Garfield (1980) and Marmor (1976), an increasing number of therapists have acknowledged the possibility that their preferred approach was not totally different from others, and that there indeed were common factors across different treatments. It is becoming more evident that these therapeutic similarities are not limited to the so-called nonspecific variables — that is, to variables for which the exact nature and specific effects are not yet known (Castonguay & Lecomte, 1989). Theoretical and, to a lesser extent, empirical investigations of the therapeutic process have identified such common factors (Castonguay, 1987; Castonguay & Lecomte, 1989; Goldfried & Padawer, 1982). These similarities have been identified within the basic structure of psychotherapy (e.g., therapeutic setting, stages), its functions (e.g., increase of hope and of a sense of mastery), and the basic process associated with the interaction (e.g., interpersonal influence, therapeutic relationship, and participants' involvement). Moreover, common factors have been identified in several aspects of communication (e.g., forms, rules, contents), in specific techniques (e.g. interpretation, paradoxical intention), as well as in more general strategies of interventions (e.g. therapist's feedback, reality testing).

This, of course, is not to say that all therapists are doing the same thing. There are unique contributions that are associated with different approaches, but these may be viewed as being potentially more complementary than was suspected 20 years ago (*see* Goldfried, 1982; Lecomte & Castonguay, 1987; Marmor & Woods, 1980; Norcross, 1986b). Complementary contributions across orientations clearly have been known to practicing clinicians, particularly when confronted with difficult clinical cases. What therapists see and do in therapy is often different than what their theories predict and suggest.

As is true for any domain of knowledge (Brown, 1977), theories of psychotherapy help us to make sense of the complex reality of human change, but at the same time prevent a fair consideration of phenomena that may be an essential part of this reality. Although one may predict that theoretical insights will continue to be important (cf., Wachtel, 1980), it is likely that the future of psychotherapy in general, and the trend toward integration in particular, will be informed by clinical research findings. For example, there exists preliminary data to suggest that if cognitive-behavior therapists would learn from interpersonally oriented psychodynamic therapists how to focus on patients' interpersonal functioning, they might improve the impact they make on patients' social adjustment. Similarly, psychodynamic therapists may be able to improve their effectiveness in bringing about symptom reduction by adopting some procedures used by cognitive-behavior therapists (Castonguay et al., 1990). Indeed, some groundbreaking steps in the integration of these two orientations currently exist, giving rise to the development of integrative clinical guidelines (Anchin, 1982; Safran & Segal, 1990).

A Focus on Specific Clinical Problems

In 1950, the first chapter ever written on psychotherapy in the *Annual Review of Psychology* (Snyder, 1950) sought to draw conclusions about psychotherapy in general. The field has become so specialized over the past four decades that it is no longer possible to address this global question. The effectiveness of psychotherapy has to be appraised with regard to specific clinical problems.

Over the years, several factors have played a role in this trend toward specificity. To begin with, the behavioral tradition of dealing with specifically defined target behaviors has resulted in a research literature that has demonstrated significant advances in clinical effectiveness for several kinds of problems, especially anxiety disorders (Barlow, 1988). The growing emphasis on DSM-based classification, receiving a major impetus from insurance companies that require its use for reimbursement purposes, has also served to underscore this problem-specific approach to intervention. Moreover, the NIMH requirement for research funding that patient populations be categorized according to DSM criteria, and that relevant therapy manuals be made available, all serve to reinforce what is likely to be a continuing trend toward specialized treatments.

One may expect that the emphasis on diversity and specification in the conceptualization and treatment of psychological disorders will increase as the field continues to mature. Considering the recent progress in process research (cf. Mahrer, 1985; Rice & Greenberg, 1984; Safran et al., 1987; Weiss & Sampson, 1986), it is very likely that for some specific disorders (e.g., depression) more energy will be spent on the specification of their psychological determinants (e.g., unresolved grief, marital conflict). This, in turn, should lead to the development of more efficient treatments. As noted in the psychotherapy chapter of a recent *Annual Review of Psychology* (Goldfried, Greenberg, & Marmar, 1990), what is needed is

> an understanding both of the determinants of any client's disorder and the mechanisms of change, and of the interventions needed to produce change for these determinants. Research must aim to demonstrate that for *this* determinant, *this* intervention produces *this* type of change process, resulting in *this* type of outcome, (p. 669)

We have come a long way since 1950.

The Use of Cognitive Science

Given the fact that different approaches to therapy acknowledge that patients' perception of self and reality contribute to their problems, we may anticipate that there will be an increasing incorporation of concepts and findings from the cognitive sciences in helping us to understand the process of therapeutic change. As more therapists receive undergraduate and graduate education that allows them to appreciate advances in the cognitive sciences, a greater number of professionals will be able to identify the potential applications of such research findings to the clinical setting. For example, the concept of "interpersonal schema," while not being associated with any given therapeutic school, nonetheless has implications for understanding such constructs as "transference" (Singer, 1988; Wachtel, 1981; Westen, 1988), and "cognitive distortions" (Beck, 1976). To the extent that such key therapeutic constructs are tied to basic research, they may be modified to increase their therapeutic effectiveness.

The Integration of Psychotherapy and Pharmacotherapy

The competition across different schools of thoughts may be replaced by one between biological psychiatry and psychosocial interventions. Although this is not the place to consider the reasons for the shift within psychiatry toward biological conceptualizations and treatments, there is every reason to believe that this trend will continue for the foreseeable future. As a result, the consumer of mental health services is confronted with these two seemingly opposing alternatives. Given the power of both psychological and physiological determinants of behavior—nurture and nature—it is unlikely that either of these two approaches is going to demonstrate unequivocal superiority. Indeed, the findings on the NIMH collaborative treatment for depression has demonstrated that, for the most part, this comparability is the case (Elkin et al., 1989).

There seems to be a growing trend in the direction of integrating psychotherapy and pharmacotherapy (Beitman & Klerman, 1991). In 1990, the NIMH sponsored a workshop to deal with the evaluation of the current status and future directions in combining both approaches for various psychological problems (B. Wolfe, personal communication, January 23, 1991). A group of clinical researchers who were actively involved in the treatment of various disorders (e.g., anxiety, depression, autism, attention deficit disorder, schizophrenia) were convened to help facilitate collaborative studies on the comparative effectiveness of the two approaches, and also the way they may be combined to enhance clinical effectiveness. Such collaborative efforts between psychosocially and biologically based professionals will very likely lead to significant progress toward the realization of our common goals, namely, the prevention and amelioration of psychological suffering.

WHERE IS PSYCHOTHERAPY INTEGRATION HEADING IN THE FUTURE?

Once a latent theme, interest in the integration of the psychotherapies has become a more active area of interest, and indeed has more recently achieved the status of a movement (Goldfried & Newman, 1992). In its most general sense, psychotherapy integration has recently been defined by Arkowitz (1992) as follows:

> Psychotherapy integration includes various attempts to look beyond the confines of single-school approaches in order to see what can be learned from other perspectives. It is characterized by an openness to various ways of integrating diverse theories and techniques. (Arkowitz, 1992, p. 262)

An increasing number of articles, chapters, and books deal directly with this topic, and the formation in 1983 of the Society for the Exploration of Psychotherapy Integration (SEPI) was a response to this growing interest.[1]

For many clinicians and researchers, the psychotherapy integration movement has been based on the possibility of combining the best of differing orientations, so that more complete theoretical models can be articulated, and more efficient treatments developed. Although there have been attempts to provide integrated therapeutic systems, most of these have tended to be somewhat limited. As psychotherapy integration becomes more a part of the mainstream, it will need to meet certain expectations that have been put forth for existing approaches, such as the need for a clearer conceptual model of change mechanisms, the availability of a research literature, and a specification of procedures within the context of therapy manuals.

Among the issues that will be predominant in the future of psychotherapy integration is the extent to which the crucial change processes are common or unique to different approaches. Although many common factors have been identified in the literature, it is possible to raise questions about their relative therapeutic importance. For example, while we may assume that the therapeutic alliance is a crucial factor in the change process, the extent to which it is sufficient to account for our therapeutic successes and failures is not clear. Further work on this question will be forthcoming. In the next few decades, those interested in psychotherapy integration will also empirically address the effectiveness of eclectic or integrative methods of treatment. There have been some recent promising attempts to provide more specific integrative therapeutic prescriptions for certain kinds of clinical problems under certain types of conditions (e.g., Beutler & Clarkin, 1990), and much more will be done on this topic.

The attempt that psychotherapy integration will make to provide the field with more valid theories and effective interventions will be characterized by the use of both top-down and bottom-up investigation strategies (Goldfried & Safran, 1986). The top-down strategy will work on the development of integrative conceptualizations of therapy that will delineate important change mechanisms drawn from clinical experience. An example of this is Wachtel's concept of *cyclical psychodynamics* (Wachtel & McKinney, 1992), referring to patients' tendencies to misperceive their relationships with others in such a way that their actions result in self-fulfilling prophecies. Practicing clinicians, regardless of orientation, can readily attest to the centrality of such a construct.

The bottom-up strategy, on the other hand, is based on empirical investigations of the change process. Significant therapeutic interactions reflecting certain key theoretical constructs will be studied (e.g., transference interpretations, disconfirmation of distorted beliefs). Such constructs will be progressively refined as more clinical manifestations are observed and analyzed. Research will also be conducted to demonstrate the interrelationship between such processes and therapeutic outcome. Findings from these studies will then be compiled and, at some point in the future, will be put together into more comprehensive integrative treatment procedures.

Top-down and bottom-up approaches to psychotherapy integration are not necessarily mutually exclusive. However, one should be aware that these strategies are closely related to basic epistemological differences among major therapy orientations (Bouchard & Guerette, 1991). As suggested by Castonguay (1989), psychodynamic, humanistic, and behavior therapists differ in what they define as valid forms of knowledge (e.g., subjective inference, felt meaning, objective observation) and in what they accept as appropriate methods to acquire such knowledge (e.g., interpretation, phenomenological exploration, experimental method). Because such diverse assumptions are based on different visions of reality and dictate different ways of reasoning, they determine, in part, why therapists from various orientations differentially formulate, explain, and treat clients' problems (Messer & Winokur, 1980). As the psychotherapy integration movement becomes more sensitive to recent developments in the philosophy of science (e.g. Brown, 1977; Mahoney, 1985, 1991), more attention will be given to epistemological issues in the understanding of change processes. The most important of these issues that need to be addressed is the potential complementarity among different epistemological assumptions. We need to know if multiple dimensions of certain mechanisms of change can be best explored by simultaneously using an empirical, hermeneutic, and phenomenological method of inquiry. Put in another way, we need to know if some kind of epistemological eclecticism is conceivable (Castonguay, 1989).

The integration movement in general, and SEPI in particular, will not only support the efforts of those professionals interested in the integration of the therapies, but will also serve a consciousness-raising function for therapists who continue to work within a given orientation. Thus, while continuing to maintain their identity according to a given school of thought, and without any active involvement in the integration movement, more therapists will nonetheless start to acknowledge the limitations of their own particular paradigm. By broadening the way they conceptualize cases, and by being more willing to experiment with other methods, such therapists will become *de facto* integrationists.

THE CONTRIBUTIONS OF THE INTEGRATION MOVEMENT TO PSYCHOTHERAPY

It is doubtful that the integration movement will provide the field with one grand theoretical integration. Given the epistemological differences already alluded to, it is hardly likely that this is possible. As long as there exist theoreticians, it is likely that there will always be competing theories.

On the other hand, one may expect that integrative efforts will lead to some consensus on intervention strategies associated with certain clinical problems. This can currently be observed with regard to certain disorders, such as pathological grief. Although theoretical conceptualizations of the change process with this problem can be psychoanalytic (Horowitz, 1976), behavioral (Callahan & Burnette, 1989), or experiential (Korb, Gorrell & Van De Riet, 1989) in nature, the clinical procedures all reflect the strategy of helping patients get in touch with the thoughts and emotions associated with the loss. Thus, continued work on integration has the potential to allow clinicians to ultimately arrive at some consensus as to how to proceed — hopefully buttressed by research to demonstrate the efficacy of these methods — even though there may be differences in the attempt to explain why these procedures are effective.

Toward the goal of fostering work on integrative psychotherapy, the NIMH workshop on research in this area (Wolfe & Goldfried, 1988) suggested that desegregation research be conducted prior to controlled outcome trials on integrative therapies. The idea is to study pure form or brand name therapies to learn more about their active mechanisms of change. In doing so, however, it will be important to determine whether or not the mechanisms of change identified by *other* forms of treatment have any relevance to the process and outcome of the particular therapy studied. The field is beginning to see such a conceptual cross-fertilization in studying the process of change.

Thus, although the concept of client "experiencing" is derived from experiential therapy (Gendlin, 1962), it has been used to determine the immediate impact of interpretations within the context of psychodynamic treatment (Silberschatz, Fretter & Curtis, 1986). The ultimate goal, of course, is to combine the interventions and processes that have been shown to have a positive impact into potentially more effective treatment procedures. The closer the integration movement gets to this goal, the better it will be for the field of psychotherapy as a whole.

Work on integrative therapy can help psychotherapy in general by sensitizing it to the communication obstacles created by each orientation's idiosyncratic jargon. To deal with this issue, the NIMH conference on psychotherapy integration research has recommended that the vernacular be considered as one potential means for communciation across orientations (Wolfe & Goldfried, 1988). However cumbersome it may be to translate key theoretical constructs into ordinary English, this somewhat awkward way of communicating with therapists of other orientations certainly would be an advance over the total inability to dialogue.

CONCLUDING COMMENTS

Although one generally cannot put too much faith in any predictions about psychotherapy, there is no doubt that the interest in the integration movement will continue to increase. The reason for such growing attraction resides in the two main objectives of the movement: 1) to achieve a more comprehensive understanding of change processes, and 2) to provide more effective intervention procedures. If integrationists are to meet their first objective, it will be by using both top-down and bottom-up investigation strategies. Significant advances in conceptualizing the mechanisms of change will be made if the constructs studied remain close to clinical experience, are formulated in a language that can be understood by all therapists, and can be influenced by basic research findings (e.g., cognitive psychology). Even more progress may be achieved if the therapeutic change process can be systematically investigated from various epistemological perspectives.

If the integration movement is to improve the therapist's repertoire with more comprehensive and effective methods, research will have to be conducted on the common and unique mechanisms of change in the treatment of specific clinical problems. Furthermore, process and outcome studies of both "pure" and "integrative" forms of interventions will have to be complemented by research findings on the determinants of specific clinical disorders. Thus, depressed patients will be approached quite differently depending upon whether their symptomatology is related to a pathological grief reaction, marital conflict, lack of interpersonal skills, inability to identify or express their emotions, or a host of other potential factors. As astutely suggested by Arkowitz (1990), knowledge of psychopathology will provide us with information about *what* needs to be changed, whereas our understanding of the change process will tell us *how* change can occur.

SUMMARY

This final chapter has considered the future of psychotherapy in general, and psychotherapy integration in particular. We may expect that psychotherapy in general will witness a consolidation of more traditional orientations; be more open toward other approaches; focus on interventions for specific clinical problems; apply findings from the cognitive sciences; and integrate psychotherapy and pharmacotherapy. We can also expect that common and unique change processes across orientations will be delineated and the effectiveness of integrative interventions will be empirically demonstrated. Although integrative psychotherapy is unlikely to provide a grand theoretical synthesis, it nonetheless can help the field to achieve a consensus on integrative strategies for certain clinical problems, foster a dialogue in a theoretically neutral language, and encourage cross-fertilization in studying the process of change.

[1]For further information about SEPI, contact: Dr. George Stricker, The Derner Institute. Adelphi University, Garden City, NY 11530.

References

Abelson, R. P. (1981). Psychological status of the script concept. *American Psychologist, 36,* 715-729.

Abramson, L. Y., Seligman, M. E. P., & Teasdale, J. D. (1978). Learned helplessness in humans: Critique and reformulation. *Journal of Abnormal Psychology, 87,* 49-74.

Addis, M. E., & Jacobson, N. S. (1991). Integration of cognitive therapy and behavioral marital therapy for depression. *Journal of Psychotherapy Integration, 1,* 249-264.

Adler, A. (1930). Individual psychology. In C. Murchinson (Ed.), *Psychologies of 1930.* Worcester, MA: Clark University Press.

Agras, W. S. (1967). Transfer during systematic desensitization therapy. *Behaviour Research and Therapy, 5,* 193-199.

Alexander, F. (1963). The dynamics of psychotherapy in light of learning theory. *American Journal of Psychiatry, 120,* 440-448.

Alexander, F., & French, T. M. (1946). *Psychoanalytic therapy: principles and application.* New York: Ronald Press.

Anchin, J. C. (1982). Sequence, pattern, and style: Integration and treatment implications of some interpersonal concepts. In J. C. Anchin & D. J. Kiesler (Eds.), *Handbook of interpersonal psychotherapy* (pp. 95-131). Elmsford, NY: Pergamon.

Anchin, J. C. (1987). Functional analysis and the social-interactional perspective: Toward an integration in the behavior change enterprise. *Journal of Integrative and Eclectic Psychotherapy, 6,* 387-399.

Appelbaum, S. A. (1975). The idealization of insight. *International Journal of Psychoanalytic Psychotherapy, 4,* 272-302.

Appelbaum, S. A. (1976). A psychoanalyst looks at gestalt therapy. In C. Hatcher & P. Himmelstein (Eds.), *The handbook of gestalt therapy.* New York: Jason Aronson.

Applebaum, S. A. (1979). *Out in inner space: A psychoanalyst explores the new therapies.* Garden City, NY: Anchor.

Arnkoff, D. B. (1983). Common and specific factors in cognitive therapy. In M. J. Lambert (Ed.), *Psychotherapy and patient relationships* (pp. 85-89). Homewood, IL: Dorsey.

251

Arkowitz, H. (November 1978, Chair). *Behavior therapy and psychoanalysis: Compatible or incompatible.* Symposium presented at the Convention of the Association for Advancement of Behavior Therapy, Chicago.

Arkowitz, H. (1990). The role of theory in psychotherapy integration. *Journal of Integrative and Eclectic Psychotherapy, 8,* 8–16.

Arkowitz, H. (1992). Integrative theories of therapy. In D. Freedheim (Ed.), *The history of psychotherapy: A century of change.* Washington, DC: APA.

Arkowitz, H., & Messer, S. B. (Eds.) (1984). *Psychoanalytic and behavior therapy: Is integration possible?* New York: Plenum.

Baer, D. M., & Stolz, S. B. (1978). A description of the Erhard Seminars Training (est) in the terms of behavior analysis. *Behaviorism, 6,* 45–70.

Bandura, A. (1961). Psychotherapy as a learning process. *Psychological Bulletin, 58,* 143–159.

Bandura, A. (1965). Behavioral modifications through modeling procedures. In L. Krasner & L. P. Ullmann (Eds.), *Research in behavior modification* (pp. 310–340). New York: Holt, Rinehart, & Winston.

Bandura, A. (1969). *Principles of behavior modification.* New York: Holt, Rinehart, & Winston.

Bandura, A. (1977). Self-efficacy: Toward a unifying theory of behavior change. *Psychological Review, 84,* 191–215.

Bandura, A. (1978). Reflections on self-efficacy. *Advances in Behaviour Research and Therapy, 1,* 237–269.

Bandura, A. (1986). *Social foundations of thought and action.* Englewood Cliffs, NJ: Prentice-Hall.

Bandura, A., & Adams, N. E. (1977). Analysis of self-efficacy theory of behavior change. *Cognitive Therapy and Research, 1,* 287–308.

Bandura, A., Adams, N. E., & Beyer, J. (1977). Cognitive processes mediating behavioral change. *Journal of Personality and Social Psychology, 35,* 125–139.

Bandura, A., Grusec, J. E., & Menlove, F. (1967). Vicarious extinction of avoidance behavior. *Journal of Personality and Social Psychology, 5,* 16–23.

Bandura, A., & Schunk, D. H. (1980). *Cultivating competence: Self-efficacy, and intrinsic interest through proximal self-motivation.* Unpublished manuscript, Stanford University.

Bandura, A., & Walters, R. H. (1963). *Social learning and personality development.* New York: Holt, Rinehart, & Winston.

Bannister, D., & Fransella, F. (1971). *Inquiring man.* Middlesex, England: Penguin Books.

Barber, J. P., & Luborsky, L. (1991). A psychodynamic view of simple phobias and prescriptive matching : A commentary. *Psychotherapy, 28,* 469–472.

Barlow, D. H. (1988). *Anxiety and its disorders: The nature and treatment of anxiety and panic.* New York: Guilford.

Barlow, D. H., & Wolfe, B. E. (1981). Behavioral approaches to anxiety disorders: A report on the NIMH-SUNY, Albany Research Conference. *Journal of Consulting and Clinical Psychology, 49,* 448-454.

Beach, S. R. H., Sandeen, E. E., & O'Leary, K. D. (1990). *Depression in marriage: A model for etiology and treatment.* New York: Guilford.

Beck, A. T. (1967).*Depression: Clinical, experimental, and theoretical aspects.* New York: Harper & Row.

Beck, A. T. (1970). Cognitive therapy: Nature and relation to behavior therapy. *Behavior Therapy, 1,* 184-200.

Beck, A. T. (1976).*Cognitive therapy and the emotional disorders.* New York: International Universities Press.

Beck, A.T. (1983). Cognitive therapy of depression: New perspectives. In P. Clayton (Ed.), *Treatment of depression* (pp. 265-290). New York: Raven.

Beck, A. T. (1985). Cognitive therapy, behavior therapy, psychoanalysis, and pharmacotherapy: A cognitive continuum. In M. J. Mahoney, & A. Freeman (Eds.), *Cognition and psychotherapy* (pp. 325-347). New York: Plenum.

Beck, A. T., & Emery, G. (1985). *Anxiety and phobias: A cognitive approach.* New York: Basic Books.

Beck, A. T., Freeman, A., & Associates (1990). *Cognitive therapy of personality disorders.* New York: Guilford Press.

Beck, A. T., Rush, A., Shaw, B., & Emery, G. (1979). *Cognitive therapy of depression.* New York: Guilford.

Beck. A. T., & Weishaar, M. (1989). Cognitive therapy. In A. Freeman, K. Simon, L. Beutler, & H. Arkowitz (Eds.), *Comprehensive handbook of cognitive therapy.* New York: Plenum.

Beech, H. R. (1960). The symptomatic treatment of writer's cramp. In H. J. Eysenck (Ed.), *Behavior therapy and the neuroses* (pp. 349-372). New York: Pergamon.

Beitman, B. D., & Klerman, G. (1991). *Integrating pharmacotherapy and psychotherapy.* Washington, D.C.: American Psychiatric Press.

Benjamin, L. S. (1982). Use of structural analysis of social behavior (SASB) to guide interventions in psychotherapy. In J. Anchin & D. Kiesler (Eds.), *Handbook of interpersonal psychotherapy* (pp. 190-212). Elmsford, NY: Pergamon.

Bergin, A. E. (1970). A note on dream changes following desensitization. *Behavior Therapy, 1,* 546-549.

Bergin, A. E. (1971). The evaluation of therapeutic outcomes. In A. E. Bergin & S. L. Garfield (Eds.), *Handbook of psychotherapy and behavior change.* New York: Wiley.

Bergin, A. E. (August 1981, Chair). *Toward a systematic eclectic therapy.*

Symposium presented at the meeting of the American Psychological Association, Los Angeles.

Bergin, A. E. (1982). The search for a psychotherapy of value. *Tijdschrist voor Psychotherapie (Journal of Psychotherapy, Amsterdam,) 8.*

Bergin, A. E., & Lambert, M. J. (1978). The evaluation of therapeutic outcomes. In S. L. Garfield & A. E. Bergin (Eds.), *Handbook of psychotherapy and behavior change: An empirical analysis. (2nd ed.).* New York: Wiley.

Bergin, A. E., & Strupp, H. H. (1972). *Changing frontiers in the science of psychotherapy.* Chicago: Aldine-Atheron.

Beutler, L. E., & Clarkin, J. (1990). *Differential treatment assignment: Toward prescriptive psychological treatments.* New York: Brunner/Mazel.

Beutler, L. E., & Consoli, A. J. (1992). Systematic eclectic psychotherapy. In J. C. Norcross & M. R. Goldfried (Eds.), *Handbook of psychotherapy integration* (pp. 264-299). New York: Basic Books.

Beutler, L. E., Engle, D., Mohr, D., Daldrup, R. J., Bergan, J., Meredith, K., & Merry, W. (1991). Predictors of differential and self-directed psychotherapeutic procedures. *Journal of Consulting and Clinical Psychology, 59,* 333-340.

Bieber, I. (1974). The concept of irrational belief systems as primary elements of psychopathology. *Journal of the American Academy of Psychoanalysis, 2,* 91-100.

Birk, L. (1970). Behavior Therapy: Integration with dynamic psychiatry. *Behavior Therapy, 1,* 522-526.

Birk, L. (1973). Psychoanalysis and behavioral analysis: Natural resonance and complementarity. *International Journal of Psychiatry, 11,* 160-166.

Birk, L. (1974). Intensive group therapy: An effective behavioral-psychoanalytic method. *American Journal of Psychiatry, 131,* 160-166.

Birk, L., & Brinkley-Birk, A. (1974). Psychoanalysis and behavior therapy. *American Journal of Psychiatry, 131,* 499-510.

Bond, I. K., & Hutchson, H. C., (1960). Application of reciprocal inhibition therapy to exhibitionism. *Canadian Medical Association Journal, 83,* 23-25.

Bordin, E. (1979). The generalizability of psychoanalytic concept of the working alliance. *Psychotherapy, 16,* 252-260.

Borkovec, T. D. (1978). Self-efficacy: Cause or reflection of behavioral change? Advances in *Behaviour Research and Therapy, 1,* 163-170.

Bouchard, M. A., & Derome, G. (1987). La Gestalt-therapie et les autres ecoles: Complementarities cliniques et perspectives de development. In C. Lecomte & L. G. Castonguay (Eds.), *Rapprochement et integration en psychotherapie: Psychanalyse, behaviorisme et humanisme* (pp. 123-156). Chicoutimi (Qc): Gaetan Morin editeur.

Bouchard, M. A., & Guerette, L. (1991). Psychotherapy as an hermeneutic experience. *Psychotherapy, 28,* 385-394.

Bower, G. H. (1975). Cognitive psychology: An introduction. In W. K. Estes

(Ed.), *Handbook of learning and cognitive processes. Vol. I: Introduction to concepts and issues.* Hillsdale, NJ: Lawrence Erlbaum Associates.

Bower, G. H. (1978). Contact of cognitive psychology with social learning theory. *Cognitive Therapy and Research, 2,* 123–146.

Bower, G. H. (1981). Mood and memory. *American Psychologist, 36,* 129–148.

Brady, J. P. (1967). Comments on methohexitone-aided desensitization. *Behaviour Research and Therapy, 5,* 259–260.

Brady, J. P. (1968). Psychotherapy by combined behavioral and dynamic approaches. *Comprehensive Psychiatry, 9,* 536–543.

Brady, J. P., Davison, G. C., Dewald, P. A., Egan G., Fadiman, J., Frank, J. D., Gill, M. M., Hoffman, I., Kempler, W., Lazarus, A. A., Raimy, V., Rotter, J. B., & Strupp, H. H. (1980). Some views on effective principles of psychotherapy. *Cognitive Therapy and Research, 4,* 269–306.

Brammer, L. M. (1969). Eclecticism revisited. *Personnel and Guidance Journal, 48,* 192–197.

Bransford, J. D., & Johnson, M. K. (1973). Consideration of some problems of comprehension. In W. G. Chase (Ed.), *Visual information processing.* New York: Academic Press.

Breger, L., & McGaugh, J. L. (1965). Critique and reformulation of "learning-theory" approaches to psychotherapy and neurosis. *Psychological Bulletin, 63,* 338–358.

Brehm, J. W., & Cohen, A. R. (1962). *Explorations in cognitive dissonance.* New York: Wiley.

Brown, H.I. (1977). *Perception, theory and commitment: The new philosophy of science.* Chicago: University of Chicago Press.

Brown, I., Jr., & Inouye, D. K. (1978). Learned helplessness through modeling: The role of perceived similarity in competence. *Journal of Personality and Social Psychology, 36,* 900–908.

Brown, M. A.(1978). Psychodynamics and behavior therapy. *Psychiatric Clinics of North America, 1,* 435–448.

Bugental, J. F. T. (1965).*The search for authenticity.* New York: Holt, Rinehart & Winston.

Burns, D. D. (1980). *Feeling good.* New York: William Morrow.

Burns, D. D. (1985). *Intimate connections.* New York: William Morrow.

Burton, A. (1976). *What makes behavior change possible?* New York: Brunner/Mazel.

Cacioppo, J. T., Glass, C. R., & Merluzzi, T. V. (1979). Self-statements and self-evaluations: A cognitive response analysis of heterosocial anxiety. *Cognitive Therapy and Research, 3,* 249–262.

Callahan, E. J., & Burnette, M. M. (1989). Intervention for pathological grieving. *The Behavior Therapist, 12,* 153–157.

Campbell, D. T., & Fiske, D. W. (1959). Convergent and discriminant validation by the multitrait-multimethod matrix. *Psychological Bulletin, 56,* 81–105.

Candiotte, M. M., & Lichtenstein, E. (1980). *Self-efficacy and relapse in smoking cessation programs.* Unpublished manuscript, University of Oregon.

Cantor, N., Mischel, W., & Schwartz, J. (1982). A prototype analysis of psychological situations. *Cognitive Psychology, 14*, 45–77.

Carroll, J. B. (1952). Ratings on traits measured by a factored personality inventory. *Journal of Abnormal and Social Psychology, 47*, 626–632.

Carroll, J. D., & Arabie, P. (1980). Multidimensional scaling. *Annual Review of Psychology, 31*, 607–649.

Carroll, J. D., & Chang, J. J. (1970). Analysis of individual differences via an N-way generalization of Eckart-Young decomposition. *Psychometricka, 15*, 283–319.

Casas, J. M. (1975). *A comparison of two mediational self-control techniques for the treatment of speech anxiety.* Unpublished doctoral dissertation, Stanford University, Stanford, CA.

Castonguay, L. G. (1987). Rapprochement en psychotherapy: Perspectives theorique, clinique et empirique. In C. Lecomte and L. G. Castonguay (Eds.), *Rapprochement et integration en psychotherapy: Psychanalyse, behaviorisme et humanisme* (pp. 3–21). Chicoutimi: Gaetan Morin.

Castonguay, L. G. (1989). Is *the logic of science also that of psychotherapy and life?* Presented at the 97th meeting of the APA, New Orleans, LA.

Castonguay, L. G., Goldfried, M. R., Hayes, A .M., Raue, P. J., Wiser, S. L., & Shapiro, D. A. (1990). *Quantitative and qualitative analyses of process-outcome data for different therapeutic approaches.* Presented at the Society for Psychotherapy Research, Wintergreen, VA.

Castonguay, L. G., & Lecomte, C. (1989). *The common factors in psychotherapy: What is known and what should be known.* Paper given at the 5th annual meeting of the Society for the Exploration of Psychotherapy Integration, San Francisco.

Cautela, J. R. (1966). A behavior therapy approach to pervasive anxiety. *Behaviour Research and Therapy, 4*, 99–109.

Cautela, J. R. (1969). Behavior therapy and self-control: *Techniques and implications. In C. M. Franks (Ed.), Behavior therapy: Assessment and status.* New York: McGraw-Hill.

Chambliss, C. A., & Murray, E. J. (1979). Efficacy attribution, locus of control, and weight loss. *Cognitive Therapy and Research, 3*, 349–353.

Chapman, L. J., & Chapman, J. P. (1969). Illusory correlations as an obstacle to the use of valid psychodiagnostic signs. *Journal of Abnormal Psychology, 74*, 271–280.

Clarke, K. M., & Greenberg, L. S. (1986). Differential effects of the gestalt two-chair intervention and problem solving in resolving decisional conflict. *Journal of Counseling Psychology, 33*, 11–15.

Cole, J. R., & Cole, S. (1973). *Social stratification in science.* Chicago: University of Chicago Press.

Crits-Cristoph, P., Baranackie, K., Kurcias, J. S., Beck, A. T., Carroll, K.,

Perry, K., Luborsky, L., McLellan, A. T., Woody, G. E., Thompson, L., Gallagher, D., & Zitrin, C. (1991). Meta-analysis of therapist effects in psychotherapy outcome studies. *Psychotherapy Research, 1*, 81–91.

Cronbach, L. J. (1956). Assessment of individual differences. *Annual Review of Psychology, 7*, 173–196.

Dahlstrom, W. G., & Welsh, G. S. (1960). *An MMPI handbook.* Minneapolis: University of Minnesota Press.

David, D. S., & Brannon, R. (Eds.) (1976). *The forty-nine percent majority: The male sex role.* Reading, MA: Addison-Wesley.

Davison, G. C. (1965). Relative contributions of differential relaxation and graded exposure to in vivo desensitization of a neurotic fear. *Proceedings of the 73rd Annual Convention of the American Psychological Association, 1*, 209–210. (Summary).

Davison, G. C. (1968). Systematic desensitization as a counterconditioning process. *Journal of Abnormal Psychology, 73*, 91–99.

Davison, G. C. (1969). Appraisal of behavior modification techniques with adults in institutional settings. In C. M. Franks (Ed.), *Behavior therapies: Assessment and appraisal.* New York: McGraw-Hill.

Davison, G. C. (1978). *Theory and practice in behavior therapy: An unconsummated marriage.* (Audiocassettes). New York: BMA Audio Cassettes.

Davison, G. C., Tsujimoto, R. N., & Glaros, A. G. (1973). Attribution and the maintenance of behavior change in falling asleep. *Journal of Abnormal Psychology, 82*, 124–133.

Davison, G. C., & Valins, S. (1968). On self-produced and drug-produced relaxation. *Behaviour Research and Therapy, 6*, 401–402.

Debus, A.G. (1966). *The English Paracelsians.* New York: Franklin Watts.

Deese, J. (1965). *The structure of associations in language and thought.* Baltimore: Johns Hopkins Press.

Dewald, P. A. (1976). Toward a general concept of the therapeutic process. *International Journal of Psychoanalytic Psychotherapy, 5*, 283–299.

Dollard, J., & Miller, N. E. (1950). *Personality and psychotherapy.* New York: McGraw-Hill.

Dryden, W. (1985). *Therapists' dilemmas.* London: Harper & Row.

D'Zurilla, T. J. (1969). Reducing heterosexual anxiety. In J. D. Kromboltz & C. E. Thoresen (Eds.), *Behavioral counseling: Cases and techniques.* New York: Holt, Rhinehart & Winston.

D'Zurilla, T. J., & Goldfried, M. R. (1971). Problem solving and behavior modification. *Journal of Abnormal Psychology, 28*, 107–126.

Egan, G. (1970). *Encounter: Group processes for interpersonal growth.* Monterey, CA.: Brooks/Cole.

Egan, G. (1973). *Face to face: The small-group experience and interpersonal growth.* Monterey, CA.: Brooks/Cole.

Egan, G. (1975). *The skilled helper.* Monterey, CA: Brooks/Cole.

Einhorn, H. J., & Hogarth, R. M. (1978). Confidence in judgment: Persistence of the illusion of validity. *Psychological Review, 85*, 395–416.

Elkin, I., Parloff, M. B., Hadley, S. W., & Autry, J. H. (1985). NIMH treatment of depression collaborative research program: Background and research plan. *Archives of General Psychiatry, 42,* 305-316.

Elkin, I. , Shea, M. T. , Watkins, J. T. , Imber, S. D., & Sotsky, S. M., et al. (1989). National Institute of Mental Health treatment of depression collaborative research program: General effectiveness of treatment. *Archives of General Psychiatry, 46,* 971-982.

Elliott, R. (1983). *Research manual for comprehensive process analysis (CPA).* Unpublished manuscript, University of Toledo.

Elliott, R., & James, E. (1989). Varieties of client experience in psychotherapy: An analysis of the literature. *Clinical Psychology Review, 9,* 443-468.

Ellis, A. (1962). *Reason and emotion in psychotherapy.* New York: Lyle Stewart.

Ellis A., & Harper, R. A. (1975). *A new guide to rational living.* Englewood Cliffs, NJ: Prentice-Hall.

Endler, N. S., & Hunt, J. McV. (1966). Sources of behavioral variance as measured by the S-R Inventory of Anxiousness. *Psychological Bulletin, 65,* 336-346.

Endler, N. S., & Hunt, J. McV.(1969). Generalizability of contributions from sources of variance in the S-R Inventories of Anxiousness. *Journal of Personality, 37,* 1-24.

Ewart, C. K., Taylor, C. B., & DeBusk, R. F. (1980). *Increasing self-efficacy after heart attack: Effects of treadmill exercise.* Paper presented at the Meeting of the American Psychological Association, Montreal.

Eysenck, H. J. (1952). The effects of psychotherapy: An evaluation. *Journal of Consulting Psychology, 16,* 319-324.

Eysenck, H. J. (1978). Expectations as causal elements in behavioural change. *Advances in Behaviour Research and Therapy, 1,* 171-175.

Fagan, J., & Shepard, I. L. (Eds.) (1970). *Gestalt therapy now.* Palo Alto, CA: Science and Behavior Books.

Fairburn, C. G. (1988). The uncertain status of the cognitive approach to bulimia nervosa. In K. M. Pirke, W. Vandereycken, & D. Ploog (Eds.), *The psychobiology of bulimia nervosa.* Berlin: Springer-Verlag.

Feather, B. W., & Rhoads, J. M. (1972a). Psychodynamic behavior therapy: I. Theory and rationale. *Archives of General Psychiatry, 26,* 496-502.

Feather, B. W., & Rhoads, J. M.(1972b). Psychodynamic behavior therapy: II. Clinical aspects. *Archives of General Psychiatry, 26,* 503-511.

Fenichel, O. (1941). Problems of psychoanalytic technique. Albany, NY: *Psychoanalytic Quarterly.*

Ferster, C. B. (1974). The difference between behavioral and conventional psychology. *The Journal of Nervous and Mental Disease, 159,* 153-157.

Fiedler, F. E. (1950). A comparison of therapeutic relationships in psychoanalytic, nondirective and Adlerian therapy. *Journal of Consulting Psychology, 14,* 436-445.

Fishbein, M., & Ajzen, I. (1975). *Belief, attitude, intention and behavior:*

An introduction to research and theory. Reading, MA: Addison-Wesley.

Fiske, S. (1982). Schema-triggered affect: Applications to social perception. In M. S. Clarke & S. T. Fiske (Eds.), *Affect and cognition: The 17th annual Carnegie symposium on cognition.* Hillside, NJ: Erlbaum.

Foa, E. B., & Emmelkamp, P. M. G. (Eds.) (1983). *Failures in behavior therapy.* New York: Wiley.

Frank, J. D. (1961). *Persuasion and healing.* Baltimore: Johns Hopkins.

Frank, J. D. (1971). Therapeutic factors in psychotherapy. *American Journal of Psychotherapy, 25,* 350–361.

Frank, J. D. (1973). *Persuasion and healing* (2nd ed.). Baltimore: John Hopkins.

Frank, J. D. (1976). Restoration of morale and behavior change. In A. Burton (Ed.), *What makes behavior change possible?* New York: Brunner/Mazel.

Frank, J. D. (1979). The present status of outcome research. *Journal of Consulting and Clinical Psychology, 47,* 310–316.

Frankl, V. E. (1965). *The doctor and the soul: From psychotherapy to logotherapy.* New York: Knopf.

Franks, C. M. (1984a). Psychoanalysis and a behavior therapy for 1983: Commentary on Leon Salzman. In H. Arkowitz & S. B. Messer (Eds.), *Psychoanalytic therapy and behavior therapy: Is integration possible?* (pp. 351–355). New York: Plenum.

Franks, C. M. (1984b). On conceptual and technical integrity in psychoanalysis and behavior therapy: Two fundamentally incompatible systems. In H. Arkowitz & S. B. Messer (Eds.), *Psychoanalytic therapy and behavior therapy: Is integration possible?* (pp. 223–247). New York: Plenum.

French, T. M. (1933). Interrelations between psychoanalysis and the experimental work of Pavlov. *American Journal of Psychiatry, 89,* 1165–1203.

Friedling C., Goldfried, M. R., & Stricker, G. (1984). Convergences in psychodynamic and behavior therapy. Paper presented at the meeting of the Eastern Psychological Association, Baltimore, MD.

Friedman, H. (1953). Perceptual regression in schizophrenia: An hypothesis suggested by use of the Rorschach test. *Journal of Projective Techniques, 17,* 171–175.

Fulkerson, S. C., & Barry, J. R. (1961). Methodology and research on the prognostic use of psychological tests. *Psychological Bulletin, 58,* 177–204.

Garber, J., & Hollon, S. D. (1980). Universal versus personal helplessness in depression: Belief in uncontrollability or incompetence? *Journal of Abnormal Psychology, 89,* 56–66.

Garfield, S. L. (1957). *Introductory clinical psychology.* New York: Macmillian.

Garfield, S. L. (1980). *Psychotherapy: An eclectic approach.* New York: Wiley.

Garfield, S. L., & Kurtz , R. (1976). Clinical psychologists in the 1970s. *American Psychologist, 31*, 1-9.

Garfield, S. L., & Kurtz, R. (1977). A study of eclectic views. *Journal of Consulting and Clinical Psychology, 45*, 78-83.

Gaston, L. (1990). The concept of the alliance and its role in psychotherapy: Theoretical and empirical consideration. *Psychotherapy, 27*, 143-153.

Geer, J. H. (1965). The development of a scale to measure fear. *Behaviour Research and Therapy, 3*, 45-53.

Geer, J. H., Davison, G. C., & Gatchel, R. J. (1970). Reduction of stress in humans through nonveridical perceived control of aversive stimulation. *Journal of Personality and Social Psychology, 16*, 731-738.

Gendlin, E. T. (1962). *Experience and the creating of meaning.* New York: The Free Press of Glencoe.

Giles, T. R. (1989). Another look at the equivalence of therapies hypotheses. *The Behavior Therapist, 12*, 174.

Glass, C. R., & Arnkoff, D.B. (1982). Thinking cognitively: Selected issues in cognitive assessment and therapy. In P.C. Kendall (Ed.), *Andvances in cognitive-behavioral research and therapy, Vol. 1* (pp. 35-71). New York: Academic Press.

Glass, C. R., & Arnkoff, D. B. (1992). Behavior therapy. In D. K. Freedheim (Ed.), *The history of psychotherapy.* Washington, DC : American Psychological Association.

Glass, D. C. (1977). *Behavior patterns, stress, and coronary disease.* Hillsdale, NJ: Erlbaum.

Glass, D. C., Singer, J. E., & Friedman, L. N. (1969). Psychic cost of adaption to an environmental stressor. *Journal of Personality and Social Psychology, 12*, 200-210.

Glasser, W. (1965). *Reality therapy: A new approach to psychiatry.* New York: Harper.

Goldfried, M. R. (1979). Anxiety reduction through cognitive-behavioral intervention. In P. C. Kendall & S. D. Hollon (Eds.), *Cognitive-behavioral interventions: Theory, research, and procedures* (pp. 117-152). New York, Academic Press.

Goldfried, M. R. (1980a). Toward the delineation of therapeutic change principles. *American Psychologist, 35*, 991-999.

Goldfried, M. R. (1980b). Psychotherapy as coping skills training. In M. J. Mahoney (Ed.), *Psychotherapy process: Current issues and future directions* (pp. 89-119). New York: Plenum.

Goldfried, M. R. (Ed.) (1982). *Converging themes in psychotherapy: Trends in psychodynamic, humanistic, and behavioral practice.* New York: Springer.

Goldfried, M. R. (1985). In vivo intervention or transference? In W. Dryden (Ed.), *Therapists' dilemmas.* London: Harper & Row.

Goldfried, M. R. (1988a).A comment on therapeutic change. *Journal of Cognitive Psychotherapy, 2*, 89-93.

Goldfried, M. R. (1988b). Application of rational restructuring to anxiety disorders. *The Counseling Psychologist, 16,* 50-68.

Goldfried, M. R. (1991). Research issues in psychotherapy integration. *Journal of Psychotherapy Integration, 1,* 5-25.

Goldfried, M. R., & Castonguay, L. G. (1993). Behavior therapy: Redefining strengths and limitations. *Behavior Therapy, 24,* 505-526.

Goldfried, M. R., Castonguay, L. G., & Safran, J. D. (1992). Core issues and future directions in psychotherapy integration. In J. C. Norcross & M. R. Goldfried (Eds.), *Handbook of psychotherapy integration* (pp. 593-616). New York: Basic Books.

Goldfried, M. R., & Davison, G. C. (1976). *Clinical behavior therapy.* New York: Holt, Rinehart & Winston.

Goldfried, M. R., & Davison, G. C. (1994). *Clinical behavior therapy (expanded edition).* New York: Wiley-Interscience.

Goldfried, M. R., Decenteceo, E. T., & Weinberg, L. (1974). Systematic rational restructuring as a self-control technique. *Behavior Therapy, 5,* 247-254.

Goldfried, M. R., & D'Zurilla, T. J. (1969). A. behavioral-analytic model for assessing competence. In C. D. Spielberger (Ed.), *Current topics in clinical and community psychology.* Vol. 1. New York: Academic Press.

Goldfried, M. R., Greenberg, L. S., & Marmar, C. (1990). Individual psychotherapy: Process and outcome. *Annual Review of Psychology, 4,* 659-688.

Goldfried, M. R., & Hayes, A. M. (1989a). Can contributions from other orientations complement behavior therapy? *The Behavior Therapist, 12,* 57-60.

Goldfried, M. R., & Hayes, A. M. (1989b). Another look at Goldfried and Hayes. *The Behavior Therapist, 12,* 174-175.

Goldfried, M. R., & Ingling, J. H. (1964). The connotative and symbolic meaning of the Bender-Gestalt. *Journal of Projective Techniques and Personality Assessment, 28,* 185-191.

Goldfried, M. R., Linehan, M. M., & Smith, J. L. (1978). The reduction of test anxiety through cognitive restructuring. *Journal of Consulting and Clinical Psychology, 46,* 32-39.

Goldfried, M. R., & Merbaum, M. (Eds.) (1973). *Behavior change through self-control.* New York: Holt, Rinehart & Winston.

Goldfried, M. R., & Newman, C.F. (1992). A history of psychotherapy integration. In J.C. Norcross and M. R. Goldfried (Eds.), *Handbook of psychotherapy integration.* New York: Basic Books.

Goldfried, M. R., Newman, C. F., & Hayes, A. M. (1989). *The coding system of therapeutic focus.* Unpublished manuscript, State University of New York at Stony Brook, Stony Brook, New York.

Goldfried, M. R., & Padawer, W. (1982). Current status and future directions in psychotherapy. In M. R. Goldfried (Ed.), *Converging themes in psychotherapy: Trends in psychodynamic, humanistic, and behavioral practice.* New York: Springer.

Goldfried, M. R., Padawer, W., & Robins, C. (1984). Social anxiety and the semantic structure of heterosocial interactions. *Journal of Abnormal Psychology, 93,* 87–97.

Goldfried, M. R., & Pomeranz, D. M. (1968). Role of assessment in behavior modification. *Psychological Reports, 23,* 75–87.

Goldfried, M. R., & Robins, C. (1983). Self-schema, cognitive bias, and the processing of therapeutic experiences. In P. C. Kendall (Ed.), *Advances in cognitive-behavioral research and therapy.* Vol. II. New York: Academic Press.

Goldfried, M. R., & Safran, J. D. (1986). Future directions in psychotherapy integration. In J. C. Norcross (Ed.), *Handbook of eclectic psychotherapy* (pp. 463–483). New York: Brunner/Mazel.

Goldfried, M. R., Stricker, G., & Weiner, I. B. (1971). *Rorschach handbook of clinical and research applications.* Englewood Cliffs, NJ : Prentice-Hall.

Goldfried, M. R., & Strupp, H. H. (November 1980). *Empirical clinical practice: A dialogue on rapprochement.* Presented at the Convention of the Association for Advancement of Behavior Therapy, New York.

Goldfried, M. R., & Trier, C. S. (1974). Effectiveness of relaxation as an active coping skill. *Journal of Abnormal Psychology, 83,* 348–355.

Goldfried, M. R., & Wachtel, P. L. (Eds.) (1983). *Newsletter of the Society for the Exploration of Psychotherapy Integration.* 1,1.

Goldfried, M. R., & Wachtel, P. L. (Eds.) (1984). *Newsletter of the Society for the Exploration of Psychotherapy Integration.* 2, 1.

Goldfried, M. R., & Wachtel, P. L. (Eds.) (1985). *Newsletter of the Society for the Exploration of Psychotherapy Integration.* 3, 1.

Goldfried, M. R., & Wachtel, P. L. (1987). Clinical and conceptual issues in psychotherapy integration: A dialogue. *Journal of Integrative and Eclectic Psychotherapy, 6,* 131–144.

Goldsamt, L. A., Goldfried, M. R., Hayes, A. M., & Kerr, S. (1992). Beck, Meichenbaum, and Strupp: A comparison of three therapies on the dimension of therapist feedback. *Psychotherapy, 29,* 167–176.

Goldstein, A. (1976). Appropriate expression training: Humanistic behavior therapy. In A. Wandersman, P. J. Poppen & D. F. Ricks (Eds.), *Humanism and behaviorism: Dialogue and growth.* Elmsford, NY: Pergamon Press.

Goldstein, A. P., Heller, K. , & Sechrest, L. B. (1966). *Psychotherapy and the psychology of behavior change.* New York: Wiley.

Goodenough, F. L. (1949). *Mental testing.* New York: Rinehart.

Gray, B. B., England, G., & Mohoney, J. L. (1965). Treatment of benign vocal nodules by reciprocal inhibition. *Behaviour Research and Therapy, 3,* 187–193.

Greenberg, L. S. (1984). A task analysis of intrapersonal conflict resolution. In L. N. Rice & L. S. Greenberg (Eds.), *Patterns of change* (pp. 67–123). New York: Guilford.

Greenberg, L. S., & Pinsof, W. M. (Eds.) (1986). *The psychotherapeutic process: A research handbook*. New York: Guilford.

Greenberg, L. S., & Safran, J. D. (1987). *Emotion in Psychotherapy*. New York: Guilford.

Greenberg, L. S., Safran, J. D. , & Rice, L. N. (1989). Experiential therapy: Its relation to cognitive therapy. In A. Freeman, K. M. Simon, L. E. Beutler, & H. Arkowitz (Eds.), *Comprehensive handbook of cognitive therapy* (pp. 169–187). New York: Plenum.

Greenberg, L. S., & Webster, M. (1982). Resolving decisional conflict by means of two-chair dialogue: Relating process to outcome. *Journal of Counseling Psychology, 29*, 468–477.

Greening, T. C. (1978). Commentary. *Journal of Humanistic Psychology, 18*, 1–4.

Greenspoon, J., & Gersten, C. D. (1967). A new look at psychological testing: Psychological testing from the standpoint of a behaviorist. *American Psychologist, 22*, 848–853.

Grinker, R. R. (1976). Discussion of Strupp's, "Some critical comments on the future of psychoanalytic therapy." *Bulletin of the Menninger Clinic, 40*, 247–254.

Guidano, V. S. (1990). *The self in process: Toward a post-rationalist cognitive therapy*. New York: Guilford.

Guidano, V. S., & Liotti, G. (1983). *Cognitive processes and emotional disorders: A structural approach to psychotherapy*. New York: Guilford.

Gurman, A. S. (1981). Integrative marital therapy: Toward the development of an interpersonal approach. In S. Budman (Ed.), *Forms of brief therapy*. New York: Guilford.

Haley, J. (1963). *Strategies of psychotherapy*. New York: Grune & Stratton.

Hamberger, K., & Lohr, J. M. (1980). Rational restructuring for anger control: A quasi-experimental case study. *Cognitive Therapy and Research, 4*, 99–102.

Hardy, G. E., & Shapiro, D. A. (1985). Therapist response modes in prescriptive vs. exploratory psychotherapy. *British Journal of Clinical Psychology, 24*, 235–245.

Hartshorne, H., & May, M. A. (1928). *Studies in the nature of character. Vol. 1. Studies in deceit*. New York: Macmillan.

Harvil, R. (1984). Bulimia: Treatment with systematic rational restructuring, response prevention, and cognitive modeling. *Journal of Counseling and Development, 63*, 250–251.

Hase, H. D., & Goldberg, L. R. (1967). Comparative validity of different strategies of constructing personality inventory scales. *Psychological Bulletin, 67*, 231–248.

Hazaleus, S. L., & Deffenbacher, J. L. (1986). Relaxation and cognitive treatments of anger. *Journal of Consulting and Clinical Psychology, 54*, 222–226.

Hebb, D. O. (1960). The American revolution. *American Psychologist, 15*, 735–745.

Henry, W. P., Schacht, T.E., & Strupp, H.H. (1990). Patient and therapist introject, interpersonal process and differential psychotherapy outcome. *Journal of Consulting and Clinical Psychology, 58,* 768-774.

Hill, C. E. (1990). Exploratory in-session process research in individual psychotherapy: A review. *Journal of Consulting and Clinical Psychology, 58,* 288-294.

Hollon, S., & Beck, A. T. (1986). Research on cognitive therapies. In S. L. Garfield & A. E. Bergin (Eds.), *Handbook of psychotherapy and behavior change* (3rd ed., pp. 443-482). New York: Wiley.

Homme, L. E. (1965). Perspectives in psychology: XXIV. Control of coverants, the operants of the mind. *Psychological Record, 15,* 501-511.

Horowitz, M. J. (1976). *Stress response syndrome.* New York: Jason Aronson.

Horwitz, L. (1976). New perspectives for psychoanalytic psychotherapy. *Bulletin of the Menninger Clinic, 40,* 263-271.

Horwitz, L. (1974). *Clinical prediction in psychotherapy.* New York: Jason Aronson.

Houts, P. S., & Serber, M. (1972). *After the turn on, what? Learning perspectives on humanistic groups.* Champaign, IL: Research Press.

Hunt, H. F. (1971). Behavioral considerations in psychiatric treatment. In J. Masserman (Ed.), *Science and psychoanalysis* (Vol. 18). New York: Grune & Stratton.

Hunt, H. F. (1976). Recurrent dilemmas in behavior therapy. In G. Serban (Ed.), *Psychopathology of human adaptation.* New York: Plenum.

Hutt, M. L. (1968). *The Hutt adaptation of the Bender-Gestalt test: Revised.* New York: Grune and Stratton.

Hutt, M. L.,& Briskin, G. J. (1960). *The clinical use of the revised Bender-Gestalt test.* New York: Grune and Stratton.

Jacobson, E. (1929). *Progressive relaxation.* Chicago: University of Chicago Press.

Jacobson, N. S., Holtzworth-Munroe, A., & Schmaling, K. B. (1989). Marital therapy and spouse involvement in the treatment of depression, agoraphobia, and alcoholism. *Journal of Consulting and Clinical Psychology, 57,* 5-10.

Jenni, M. A., & Wollersheim, J. P. (1979). Cognitive therapy, stress management training and the Type A behavior pattern. *Cognitive Therapy and Research, 3,* 61-73.

Jessor, R., & Hammond, K.R. (1957). Construct validity and the Taylor Anxiety Scale. *Psychological Bulletin, 54,* 161-170.

Johnson, W. (1946). *People in quandaries.* New York: Harper & Row.

Jones, E. E., & Nisbett, R. E. (1971). *The actor and observer: Divergent perceptions of the causes of behavior.* New York: General Learning Press.

Jung, C. G. (1910). The association method. *American Journal of Psychology, 21,* 219-269.

Kagan, J. (1956). The measurement of overt aggression from fantasy. *Journal of Abnormal and Social Psychology, 52,* 390-393.

Kanfer, F. H., & Phillips, J. S. (1966). Behavior therapy: A panacea for all ills or a passing fancy? *Archives of General Psychiatry, 15,* 114-128.

Kanfer, F. H. & Phillips, J. S. (1970). *Learning foundations of behavior therapy.* New York: John Wiley.

Kanfer, F. H., & Saslow, G. (1965). Behavior analysis: An alternative to diagnostic classification. *Archives of General Psychiatry, 12,* 529-538.

Kanfer, F. H., & Saslow, G. (1969). Behavioral diagnosis. In C. M. Franks (Ed.), *Behavior therapy: Appraisal and status.* New York: McGraw-Hill.

Kanter, N. J., & Goldfried, M. R. (1979). Relative effectiveness of rational restructuring and self-control desensitization in the reduction of interpersonal anxiety. *Behavior Therapy, 10,* 472-490.

Kaplan, H. S. (1974). *The new sex therapy.* New York: Brunner/Mazel.

Karoly, P. (1980). Person variables in therapeutic change and development. In P. Karoly & J. J. Steffen (Eds.). *Improving the long-term effects of psychotherapy* (pp. 195-261). New York: Gardner Press.

Kazdin, A.E. (1979). Imagery elaboration and self-efficacy in the covert modeling treatment of unassertive behavior. *Journal of Consulting and Clinical Psychology, 47,* 725-733.

Kazdin, A. E. (1986a). Treatment research: The investigation and evaluation of psychotherapy. In M. Hersen, A. E. Kazdin, & A. S. Bellack (Eds.), *The clinical psychology handbook* (pp. 265-284). New York: Pergamon.

Kazdin, A.E. (1986b). Comparative outcome studies of psychotherapy: Methodological issues and strategies. *Journal of Consulting and Clinical Psychology, 54,* 95-105.

Kelly, E. L., Goldberg, L. R., Fiske, D. W., & Kilkowski, J. M. (1978). Twenty-five years later: A follow-up study of the graduate students in clinical psychology assessed in the VA selection research project. *American Psychologist, 33,* 746-755.

Kelly, G. A. (1955). *The psychology of personal constructs.* New York: Norton.

Kelly, G. A. (1958). The theory and technique of assessment. In P. R. Farnsworth and Q. McNemar (Eds.), *Annual review of psychology.* (pp. 323-352). Palo Alto, CA: Annual Reviews.

Kendall, P. C. (1982). Integration: Behavior therapy and other schools of thought. *Behavior Therapy, 13,* 559-571.

Kendall, P. C., & Hollon, S. D. (Eds.) (1981). *Assessment strategies for cognitive-behavioral interventions.* New York: Academic Press.

Kendall, P. C., & Kriss, M. R. (1983). Cognitive-behavioral interventions. In C. Eugene Walker (Ed.), *Handbook of clinical psychology* (pp. 770-819). Homewood, IL: Dow Jones-Irwin.

Kerr, S., Goldfried, M. R., Hayes, A. M., & Goldsamt, L. A. (June 1989). *Differences in therapeutic focus in an interpersonal-psychodynamic and cognitive-behavioral therapy.* Paper presented at the 20th annual meeting of the Society for Psychotherapy Research, Toronto, Canada.

Kiesler, D. J. (1966). Some myths of psychotherapy research and the search for a paradigm. *Psychological Bulletin, 65,* 110-136.

Kihlstrom, J. F., & Nasby, W. (1981). Cognitive tasks in clinical assessment: An exercise in applied psychology. In P. C. Kendall & S. D. Hollon (Eds.), *Assessment strategies for cognitive-behavioral interventions.* New York: Academic Press.

Klein, M., Dittmann, A. T., Parloff, M. B., & Gill, M. M. (1969). Behavior therapy: Observations and reflections. *Journal of Consulting and Clinical Psychology, 33,* 259-266.

Klerman, G. L., Weissman, M. M., Rounsaville, B., & Chevron, E. (1984). *Interpersonal psychotherapy of depression.* New York: Basic Books.

Koerner, K., & Linehan, M. (1992). Integrative therapy for borderline personality disorder: Dialectical behavior therapy. In J. C. Norcross & M. R. Goldfried (Eds.), *Handbook of psychotherapy integration* (pp. 433-459). New York: Basic Books.

Kohlenberg, R.J., & Tsai, M. (1989). Functional analytic psychotherapy. In N.S. Jacobson (Ed.), *Psychotherapists in clinical practice* (pp. 388-443). New York: Guilford.

Kohlenberg, R. J., & Tsai, M. (1991). *Functional analytic psychotherapy.* New York: Plenum.

Korb, M. P., Gorrell, J., & Van De Riet, V. (1989). Gestalt therapy: *Practice and theory* (2nd ed.). Elmsford, NY: Pergamon Press.

Korchin, S. J., & Schuldberg, D. (1981). The future of clinical assessment. *American Psychologist, 36,* 1147-1158.

Krasner, L. (1978). The future and the past in the behaviorism-humanism dialogue. *American Psychologist, 33,* 799-804.

Kubie, L. S. (1934). Relation of the conditioned reflex to psychoanalytic technic. *Archives of Neurology and Psychiatry, 32,* 1137-1142.

Kuhn, T. S. (1970). *The structure of scientific revolutions* (2nd ed.). Chicago: University of Chicago Press.

Lambert, M. J. (1989). The individual therapist's contribution to psychotherapy process outcome. *Clinical Psychology Review, 9,* 469-485.

Lambert, M. J., Shapiro, D. A., & Bergin, A. E. (1986). The effectiveness of psychotherapy. In S. L. Garfield & A. E. Bergin (Eds.), *Handbook of psychotherapy and behavior change* (3rd ed., pp. 157-211). New York: Wiley.

Lambley, P. (1976). The use of assertive training and psychodynamic insight in the treatment of migraine headaches: A case study. *Journal of Nervous and Mental Disease, 163,* 61-64.

Landau, R. J. (1980). The role of semantic schemata in phobic word interpretation. *Cognitive Therapy and Research, 4,* 427-434.

Landau, R. J., & Goldfried, M. R. (1981). The assessment of schemata: A unifying framework for cognitive, behavioral, and traditional assessment. In P. C. Kendall & S. D. Hollon (Eds.), *Assessment strategies for cognitive-behavioral interventions* (pp. 363-399). New York: Academic Press.

Landsman, T. (August 1974). *Not an adversity but a welcome diversity*. Paper presented at the meeting of the American Psychological Association, New Orleans.

Lang, P. J. (1968). Fear reduction and fear behavior: Problems in treating a construct. In H. H. Strupp & L. Luborsky (Eds.), *Research in psychotherapy*. Washington, D.C.: American Psychological Association.

Lang, P. J. (1969). The mechanics of desensitization and the laboratory study of human fear. In C. M. Franks (Ed.), *Behavior therapy: Assessment and status*. New York: McGraw-Hill.

Lang, P. J. (1978). Self-efficacy theory: Thoughts on cognition and unification. *Advances in Behaviour Research and Therapy, 1,* 187-192.

Lang, P. J., & Lazovik, A. D. (1963). Experimental desensitization of a phobia. *Journal of Abnormal and Social Psychology, 66,* 519-525.

Lang, P. J., Lazovik, A. D., & Reynolds, D. J. (1965). Desensitization, suggestibility, and pseudotherapy. *Journal of Abnormal Psychology, 70,* 395-402.

Langer, E. J., & Rodin, J. (1976). The effects of choice and enhanced personal responsibility for the aged: A field experiment in a institutional setting. *Journal of Personality and Social Psychology, 34,* 191-198.

Larson, D. (1980). Therapeutic schools, styles, and schoolism: A national survey. *Journal of Humanistic Psychology, 20,* 3-20.

Lazarus, A. A. (1965). Behavior therapy, incomplete treatment, and symptom substitution. *Journal of Nervous and Mental Disease, 140,* 80-86.

Lazarus, A. A. (1967). In support of technical eclecticism. *Psychological Reports, 21,* 415-416.

Lazarus, A. A. (1971). *Behavior therapy and beyond*. New York: McGraw-Hill.

Lazarus, A. A. (1976). *Multimodal behavior therapy*. New York: Springer.

Lazarus, A. A. (1977). Has behavior therapy outlived its usefulness? *American Psychologist, 32,* 550-554.

Lazarus, A. A. (1981). *The practice of multimodal therapy*. New York: McGraw Hill.

Lazarus, A. A., & Davison G. C. (1971). Clinical innovation in research and practice. In A. E. Bergin & S. L. Garfield (Eds.), *Handbook of psychotherapy and behavior change*. New York: Wiley.

Lazarus, R. S., & Launier, R. (1978). Stress-related transactions between person and environment. In L. A. Pervin & M. Lewis (Eds.), *Perspectives in interactional psychology*. New York: Plenum.

Lecomte, C., & Castonguay, L. G. (Eds.) (1987). *Rapprochement et integration en psychotherapie*. Montreal: Gaetan Morin Editeur.

Lefcourt, H. M. (1976). *Locus of control: Current trends in theory and research*. Hillsdale, NJ: Erlbaum.

Leitenberg, H., Agras, W. S., Barlow, D. H., & Oliveau, D. C. (1969). Contribution of selective positive reinforcement and therapeutic instructions to systematic desensitization therapy. *Journal of Abnormal Psychology, 74,* 113-118.

Lent, R. W., Russell, R. K., & Zamostny, K. P. (1981). Comparisons of cue-controlled desensitization, rational restructuring, and a credible placebo in the treatment of speech anxiety. *Journal of Consulting and Clinical Psychology, 49,* 608–610.

Levay, A. N., Weissberg, J. H., & Blaustein, A. B. (1976). Concurrent sex therapy and psychoanalytic psychotherapy by separate therapists: Effectiveness and implications. *Psychiatry, 39,* 355–363.

Leventhal, A. M. (1968). Use of a behavioral approach within a traditional psychotherapeutic context: A case study. *Journal of Abnormal Psychology, 73,* 178–182.

Levis, D. J. (1988). Observations and experience from clinical practice: A critical ingredient for advancing behavioral theory and therapy. *The Behavior Therapist, 11,* 95–99.

Lewin, K. (1939). Field theory and experiment in social psychology: Concepts and methods. *American Journal of Sociology, 44,* 868–896.

Lewis, W. C. (1972). *Why people change.* New York: Holt, Rinehart & Winston.

Linehan, M. M. (1987). Dialectical behavioral therapy: A cognitive-behavioral approach to parasuicide. *Journal of Personality Disorders, 1,* 328–333.

Linehan, M.M. (1993). *Cognitive-behavioral treatment of borderline personality disorder.* New York: Guilford.

Linehan, M. M., Goldfried, M. R., & Goldfried, A. P. (1979). Assertion training: Skill acquisition or cognitive restructuring. *Behavior Therapy, 10,* 372–388.

Loevinger, J. (1957). Objective tests as instruments of psychological theory. *Psychological Reports, 3,* (Monograph Supplement 9).

London, P. (1964). *The modes and morals of psychotherapy.* New York: Holt, Rinehart & Winston.

London, P. (1972). The end of ideology in behavior modification. *American Psychologist, 27,* 913–920.

London, P. (1986). *The modes and morals of psychotherapy* (2nd ed.) Washington D.C.: Hemisphere Publishing Corp.

Luborsky, L. (1984). *Principles of psychoanalytic psychotherapy. A manual for supportive-expressive (SE) treatment.* New York: Basic Books.

Luborsky, L., Singer, B., & Luborsky, L. (1975). Comparative studies of psychotherapies: Is it true that "everybody has won and all must have prizes?" *Archives of General Psychiatry, 32,* 995–1008.

MacFarlane, J. W., & Tuddenham, R. D. (1951). Problems in the validation of projective techniques. In H. H. Anderson & G. L. Anderson (Eds.), *An introduction to projective techniques.* Englewood Cliffs, NJ: Prentice Hall.

Mahoney, M. J. (1974). *Cognition and behavior modification.* Cambridge, MA: Ballinger.

Mahoney, M. J. (1979). Cognitive and non-cognitive views in behavior modification. In P. O. Sjoden & S. Bates (Eds.), *Trends in behavior therapy.* New York: Plenum.

Mahoney, M. J. (1985). Psychotherapy and human change processes. In M. J. Mahoney and A. Freedman (Eds.), *Psychotherapy and cognition* (pp. 3–48). New York: Plenum.

Mahoney, M. J. (1991). *Human change processes: Theoretical bases for psychotherapy.* New York: Basic Books.

Mahoney, M. J., Norcross, J. C., Prochaska, J. O., & Missar, C. D. (1989). Psychologocial development and optimal psychotherapy: Converging perspectives among clinical psychologists. *Journal of Integrative and Eclectic Psychotherapy, 8,* 251–263.

Mahoney, M. J., & Wachtel, P. L. (May 1982). *Convergence of psychoanalytic and behavioral therapy.* Presentation at the Institute for Psychological Study, New York .

Mahrer, A. (1985). *Psychotherapeutic change: An alternative approach to meaning and measurement.* New York: Norton.

Mahrer, A., & Nadler, W. (1986). Good moments in psychotherapy: A preliminary review, a test and some promising research avenues. *Journal of Consulting and Clinical Psychology, 54,* 10–15.

Malkiewich, L. E., & Merluzzi, T. V. (1980). Rational restructuring versus desensitization with clients of diverse conceptual levels: A test of a client-treatment matching model. *Journal of Counseling Psychology, 5,* 453–461.

Marks, I. M. (1969). *Fears and phobias.* New York: Academic Press.

Marks, I. M. (1971). The future of psychotherapies. *British Journal of Psychiatry, 118,* 69–73.

Marks, I. M., & Gelder, M. G. (1966). Common ground between behavior therapy and psychodynamic methods. *British Journal of Medical Psychology, 39,* 11–23.

Markus, H. (1977). Self-schemata and processing information about the self. *Journal of Personality and Social Psychology, 35,* 63–78.

Marmor, J. (1964). Psychoanalytic therapy and theories of learning. In J. Masserman (Ed.), *Science and Psychoanalysis* (Vol. 7). New York: Grune & Stratton.

Marmor, J. (1969). Neurosis and the psychotherapeutic process: Similarities and differences in the behavioral and psychodynamic conceptions. *International Journal of Psychiatry, 7,* 514–519.

Marmor, J. (1971). Dynamic psychotherapy and behavior therapy: Are they irreconcilable? *Archives of General Psychiatry, 24,* 22–28.

Marmor, J. (1976). Common operational factors in diverse approaches to behavior change. In A. Burton (Ed.), *What makes behavior change possible?* (pp. 3–12). New York: Brunner/Mazel.

Marmor, J., & Woods, S. M. (Eds.) (1980). *The interface between psychodynamic and behavioral therapies.* New York: Plenum.

Martin, D. G. (1972). *Learning-based client centered therapy.* Monterey, CA: Brooks/Cole.

Martorano, R. D., Nietzel, M. T., & Melnick, J. (1977). *A comparison of covert modeling with reply training and systematic rational restructuring as treatment for unassertiveness.* Unpublished manuscript, University of Kentucky, Lexington.

Maslow, A. H. (1966). *The psychology of science: A reconnaissance.* New York: Harper & Row.

Masters, W. H., & Johnson, V. E. (1970). *Human sexual inadequacy.* Boston: Little, Brown.

Mavissakalian, M., & Hamman, M. S. (1987). DSM-III Personality disorder in agoraphobia: II. Changes with treatment. *Comprehensive Psychiatry, 28,* 356–361.

McFall, R. M. (1970). Effects of self-monitoring on normal smoking behavior. *Journal of Consulting and Clinical Psychology, 35,* 135–142.

Meehl, P. E. (1960). The cognitive activity of the clinician. *American Psychologist, 15,* 19–27.

Meichenbaum, D. H. (1974). *Cognitive behavior modification.* Morristown, NJ: General Learning Press.

Meichenbaum, D. H. (1977). *Cognitive behavior modification: An integrative approach.* New York: Plenum.

Meichenbaum, D. H. (1980). *Nature of conscious and unconscious processes: Issues in cognitive assessment.* Invited address presented at the meeting of the Eastern Psychological Association, Hartford, CT.

Meichenbaum, D.H., & Butler, L. (1980). Cognitive ethology: Assessing the streams of cognition and emotion. In K. Blankstein, P. Pliner, & J. Polivy (Eds.), *Advances in the study of communication and affect: Assessment and modification of emotional behavior* (Vol. 6). New York: Plenum.

Meichenbaum, D.H., & Gilmore, J. B. (1984). The nature of unconscious processes: A cognitive-behavioral perspective. In K. Bowers & D. Meichenbaum (Eds.), *The unconscious reconsidered* (pp. 273–298). New York: Wiley Interscience.

Merluzzi, T. V., Glass, C. R., & Genest, M. (Eds.) (1981). *Cognitive assessment.* New York: Guilford.

Merton, R.K. (1969). Behavior patterns of scientists. *American Scholar, 38,* 197–225.

Merton, R. K. (1970). *Science, technology, and society in seventeenth-century England.* New York: Harper & Row (originally published 1938).

Messer, S. B. (1986). Behavioral and psychoanalytic perspectives at therapeutic choice points. *American Psychologist, 41,* 1261–1272.

Messer, S. B., & Winokur, M. (1980). Some limits to the integration of psychoanalytic and behavior therapy. *American Psychologist, 35,* 818–827.

Metalsky, G. I., & Abramson, L. Y. (1981). Attributional styles: Toward a framework for conceptualization and assessment. In P. C. Kendall & S. D. Hollon (Eds.), *Assessment strategies for cognitive-behavioral interventions.* New York: Academic Press.

Meyer, V., & Crisp, A.H. (1966). Some problems of behavior therapy. *British Journal of Psychiatry, 112,* 367-382.

Michelson, L. (1986). Treatment consonance and response profiles in agoraphobia: The role of individual differences in cognitive, behavioral and physiological treatments. *Behaviour Research and Therapy, 24,* 263-275.

Mikulas, W. L. (1978). Four noble truths of Buddhism related to behavior therapy. *Psychological Record, 28,* 59-67.

Mischel, W. (1968). *Personality and assessment.* New York: Wiley.

Mischel, W. (1969). Continuity and change in personality. *American Psychologist, 24,* 1012-1018.

Mischel, W., & Ebbesen, E. B. (1970). Attention in delay of gratification. *Journal of Personality and Social Psychology, 16,* 329-337.

Mischel, W., & Peake, P. K. (1982). Beyond déjà vu in the search for cross-situational consistency. *Psychological Review, 89,* 730-755.

Mitchell, K. M., Bozarth, J. D., & Krauft, C. C. (1977). A reappraisal of the therapeutic effectiveness of accurate empathy, non-possessive warmth and genuineness. In A. S. Gurman & A. M. Razin (Eds.), *Effective psychotherapy: A handbook of research* (pp. 482-502). New York: Pergamon Press.

Moos, R. H. (1968). Behavioral effects of being observed: Reactions to a wireless radio transmitter. *Journal of Consulting and Clinical Psychology, 32,* 383-388.

Moos, R. H. (1969). Sources of variance in responses to questionnaires and in behavior. *Journal of Abnormal Psychology, 74,* 405-412.

Mowrer, O. H. (1960). Learning theory and the symbolic processes. New York: Wiley.

Mozer, M. H. (1979). Confessions of an ex-behaviorist. *The Behavior Therapist, 2,* 3.

Murphy, G. (1947). *Personality: A biosocial approach to its origins and structures.* New York: Harper & Row.

Murray, H. A. (1938). *Explorations in personality.* New York: Oxford University Press.

Murray, N. E. (1976). A dynamic synthesis of analytic and behavioral approaches to symptoms. *American Journal of Psychotherapy, 30,* 561-569.

Murstein, B. I. (1961). Assumptions, adaptation level, and projective techniques. *Perceptual and Motor Skills, 12,* 107-125.

Murstein, B. I. (1963). *Theory and research in projective techniques. (emphasizing the TAT).* New York: Wiley.

Neimeyer, G. J., & Neimeyer, R. A. (1981). Personal construct perspectives on cognitive assessment. In T. Merlussi, C. Glass, & M. Genest (Eds)., *Cognitive Assessment.* New York: Guilford.

Neisser, U. (1976). *Cognition and reality.* San Francisco: Freeman.

Nelson-Gray, R. O. (November 1991). Treatment matching for unipolar depression. In M. E. Addis (Chair), *Matching clients to treatments: Clinical and research considerations*. Symposium conducted at the meeting of the Association for Advancement of Behavior Therapy, New York.

Nielson, A. C. (1980). Gestalt and psychoanalytic therapies: Structural analysis and rapprochement. *American Journal of Psychotherapy, 34*, 534–544.

Nobel, C. E. (1952). An analysis of meaning. *Psychological Review, 59*, 421–430.

Norcross, J. C. (1986a). Eclectic psychotherapy: An introduction and overview. In J. C. Norcross (Ed.), *Handbook of eclectic psychotherapy* (pp. 3–24). New York: Brunner/Mazel.

Norcross, J. C. (Ed.) (1986b). *Handbook of eclectic psychotherapy*. New York: Brunner/Mazel.

Norcross, J. C. (1988). The exclusivity myth and the equifinality principle in psychotherapy. *Journal of Integrative and Eclectic Psychotherapy, 7*, 415–421.

O'Leary, K. D. (1984). The image of behavior therapy: It is time to take a stand. *Behavior Therapy, 15*, 219–233.

O'Leary, K. D., & Turkewitz, H. (1978). Marital therapy from a behavioral perspective. In T. J. Paolino & B. S. McCrady (Eds.), *Marriage and marital therapy: Psychoanalytic, behavioral, and systems theory perspectives*. New York: Brunner/Mazel.

O'Leary, K. D., & Wilson, G. T. (1987). *Behavior therapy: Application and outcome* (2nd ed.). New York: Prentice-Hall.

Orlinsky, D. E., & Howard, K. I. (1986). Process and outcome in psychotherapy. In S. L. Garfield & A. E. Bergin (Eds.), *Handbook of psychotherapy and behavior change* (3rd ed., pp. 311–381). New York: Wiley.

Osarchuk, M. (1974). *A comparison of a cognitive, a behavior therapy and cognitive plus behavior therapy treatment of test anxious college students*. Unpublished doctoral dissertation, Adelphi University, Garden City, NY.

Osgood, C. E. (1953). *Method and theory in experimental psychology*. New York: Oxford University Press.

Osgood, C. E., Suci, G. J., & Tannenbaum, P. H. (1957). *The measurement of meaning*, Urbana, IL: University of Illinois Press.

Parloff, M. B. (1976). Shopping for the right therapy. *Saturday Review*, February 21, pp.14–16.

Parloff, M. B. (1979). Can psychotherapy research guide the policy maker? A little knowledge may be a dangerous thing. *American Psychologist, 34*, 296–306.

Parsons, T. (1951). *The social system*. New York: Free Press.

Patterson, C. H. (1967). Divergence and convergence in psychotherapy. *American Journal of Psychotherapy, 21*, 4–17.

Patterson, G. R., & Forgatch, M. S. (1985). Therapist behavior as a determinant for client non-compliance: A paradox for the behavior modifier. *Journal of Consulting and Clinical Psychology, 53*, 846–851.

Patterson, G. R., & Harris, A. (September 1968). *Some methodological considerations for observation procedures.* Paper presented at the meeting of the American Psychological Association, San Francisco.

Paul, G.L. (1966). *Insight vs. desensitization in psychotherapy.* Stanford: Stanford University Press.

Paul, G. L. (1967). Strategy of outcome research in psychotherapy. *Journal of Consulting Psychology, 31,* 109-119.

Paul, G. L., & Shannon, D. T. (1966). Treatment of anxiety through systematic desensitization in therapy groups. *Journal of Abnormal Psychology, 71,* 124-135.

Perls, F. (1973). *The gestalt approach and eye witness therapy.* Palo Alto, CA: Science and Behavior Books, Bantam Edition.

Persons, J.B. (1989). *Cognitive therapy in practice: A case formulation approach.* New York: Norton.

Peterson, D. R. (1968). *The clinical study of social behavior.* New York: Appleton-Century-Crofts.

Phares, R. J. (1976). *Locus of control in personality.* Morristown, NJ: General Learning Press.

Polster, E., & Polster, M. (1973). *Gestalt therapy integrated.* New York: Brunner/Mazel.

Pretzer, J., & Fleming, B. (1989). Cognitive-behavioral treatment of personality disorders. *The Behavior Therapist, 12,* 105-109.

Prochaska, J. O. (1979). *Systems of psychotherapy: A transtheoretical analysis.* Homewood, IL: Dorsey.

Prochaska, J. O., & DiClemente, D. C. (1984). *The transtheoretical approach: Crossing the traditional boundaries of therapy.* Homewood, IL: Dow Jones-Irvin.

Rachman, S. (1965). Studies in desensitization — 1: The separate effects of relaxation and desensitization. *Behaviour Research and Therapy, 3,* 245-251.

Rachman, S. (1978). Perceived self-efficacy: Analyses of Bandura's theory of behavioral change. *Advances in Behaviour Research and Therapy, 1,* 139-269.

Raimy, V. (1975). *Misunderstandings of the self.* San Francisco: Jossy-Bass.

Raimy, V. (1976). Changing misconceptions as the therapeutic task. In A. Burton (Ed.), *What makes behavior change possible?* New York: Brunner/Mazel.

Raue, P. J., Castonguay, L. G., & Goldfried, M. R. (1993). The working alliance: A comparison of two therapies. *Psychotherapy Research, 3,* 197-207.

Raue, P. J., & Goldfried, M. R. (1994). The therapeutic alliance in cognitive-behavior therapy. In A. O. Horvath & L. S. Greenberg (Eds.), *The working alliance: Theory, research, and practice.* New York: Wiley.

Rehm. L. P., & Marston, A. R. (1968). Reduction of social anxiety through modification of self-reinforcement: An instigation therapy technique. *Journal of Consulting and Clinical Psychology, 32,* 565-574.

Reich, W. (1949). *Character analysis* (T. P. Wolfe, Trans.). New York: Orgone Institute Press. (Originally published, 1933).

Reid, W. (1987). Psychanalyse et/ou behaviorisme. In C. Lecomte and L. G. Castonguay (Eds.), Rapprochement et integration en psychotherapie: Psychoanalyse, behaviorisme et humanisme (pp. 51-61). Chicoutimi (Qc): Gaetan Morin editeur.

Rhoads, J. M. (1981). The integration of behavior therapy and psychoanalytic theory. *Journal of Psychiatric Treatment and Evaluation, 3*, 1-6.

Rhoads, J. M., & Feather, B. W. (1974). The application of psychodynamic to behavior therapy. *American Journal of Psychiatry, 131*, 17-20.

Rice, L. N. (1980). *The context of recurring events during psychotherapy: A task analysis of an event from client-centered therapy*. Paper presented at the meetings of the Society for Psychotherapy Research, Asilomar, CA.

Rice, L. N., & Greenberg L. S. (Eds.) (1984). *Patterns of change: Intensive analysis of psychotherapy process*. New York: Guilford.

Ricks, D. F., Wandersman, A., & Poppen, P. J. (1976). Humanism and behaviorism: Toward new syntheses. In A. Wandersman, P. J. Poppen, & D. F. Ricks (Eds.), *Humanism and behaviorism: Dialogue and growth*. Elmsford, N.Y. Pergamon Press.

Robertson, M. (1979). Some observations from an eclectic therapist. *Psychotherapy: Theory, Research, and Practice, 16*, 18-21.

Rodin, J., & Langer, E. J. (1977). Long-term effects of a control-relevant intervention with the institutionalized aged. *Journal of Personality and Social Psychology, 35*, 897-902.

Rogers, C. R. (1951). *Client-centered therapy*. Boston: Houghton Mifflin.

Rogers, C. R. (1957). The necessary and sufficient conditions of therapeutic personality change. *Journal of Consulting Psychology, 21*, 95-103.

Rogers, C. R. (1963). Psychotherapy today or where do we go from here? *American Journal of Psychotherapy, 17*, 5-15.

Rogers, C. R., & Skinner, B.F. (1956). Some issues concerning the control of human behavior. *Science, 124*, 1057-1066.

Rosenberg, S. (1977). New approaches to the analysis of personal constructs in person perception. In J. K. Cole & A. W. Landfield (Eds.), *Nebraska Symposium on Motivation*, 24, (pp. 174-242). Lincoln: University of Nebraska Press.

Rosenthal, T. L. (1978). Bandura's self-efficacy theory: Thought *is* father to the deed. *Advances in Behaviour Research and Therapy, 1*, 203-209.

Rosenzweig, S. (1936). Some implicit common factors in diverse methods in psychotherapy. *American Journal of Orthopsychiatry, 6*, 412-415.

Ross, L. (1977). The intuitive psychologist and his shortcomings: Distortions in the attribution process. In L. Berkowiz (Ed.), *Advances in experimental social psychology* (Vol. 10). New York: Academic Press.

Ross, L., Lepper, M. & Hubbard, M. (1975). Perseverance in self-perception and social perception: Biased attributional processes in the debriefing paradigm. *Journal of Personality and Social Psychology, 32*, 880-892.

Rotter, J. B. (1954). *Social learning and clinical psychology*. Englewood Cliffs, NJ: Prentice-Hall.

Rotter, J. B. (1960). Some implications of a social learning theory for the prediction of goal directed behavior from testing situations. *Psychological Review, 67*, 301–316.

Rush, A. J., & Shaw, B. F. (1983). Failures in treating depression by cognitive therapy. In E. B. Foa & P. G. M. Emmelkamp (Eds.), *Failures in behavior therapy* (pp. 217–228). New York: Wiley.

Ryle, A. A. (1978). A common language for the psychotherapies? *British Journal of Psychiatry, 132*, 585–594.

Ryle, A. A. (1980). *Integrating opposing theories in a cognitive model of neurotic problems*. Unpublished manuscript, University of Sussex.

Ryle, A. A. (1987). Cognitive psychology as a common language for psychotherapy. *Journal of Integrative and Eclectic Psychotherapy, 6*, 168–172.

Safran, J. D. (1990a). Towards a refinement of cognitive therapy in light of interpersonal theory: I. *Clinical Psychology Review, 10*, 87–105.

Safran, J. D. (1990b). Towards a refinement of cognitive therapy in light of interpersonal theory: II. Practice. *Clinical Psychology Review, 10*, 107–121.

Safran, J. D., Crocker, P. M. , McMain, S., & Murray, P. (1990). Therapeutic alliance rupture as a therapy event for empirical investigations. *Psychotherapy, 27*, 154–165.

Safran, J. D., & Greenberg, L. S. (1986). Hot cognition and psychotherapy process: An information-processing/ecological approach. In P. C. Kendall (Ed.) *Advances in cognitive-behavioral research and therapy* (Vol. 5) (pp. 143–177). New York: Academic.

Safran, J. D., & Segal, Z. V. (1990). *Interpersonal process in cognitive therapy.* New York: Basic Books.

Safran, J. D., Vallis, T, M., Segal, Z. V., Shaw, B. F., Balog, W., & Epstein, L. (1987). Measuring session change in cognitive therapy. *Journal of Cognitive Psychotherapy: An International Quarterly, 1*, 117–128.

Salzman, L. (1984). The behavioral scientist as integrator: Commentary on Cyril M. Franks. In H. Arkowitz & S. Messer (Eds.), *Psychoanalytic therapy and behavior therapy: Is integration possible?* (pp. 249–252). New York: Plenum.

Sarason, I. G. (1979). Three lacunae of cognitive therapy. *Cognitive Therapy and Research, 3*, 223–235.

Segraves, R. T., & Smith, R. C. (1976). Concurrent psychotherapy and behavior therapy: Treatment of psychoneurotic outpatients. *Archives of General Psychiatry, 33*, 756–763.

Schachter, S., & Singer, J. E. (1962). Cognitive, social, and physiological determinants of emotional state. *Psychological Review, 69*, 379–399.

Schank, R. C., & Abelson, R. P. (1977). *Scripts, plans, goals, and understanding*. Hillsdale, NJ: Erlbaum.

Schindler, L., Hohenberger-Sieber, E., & Hahlweg, K. (1989). Observing client-therapist interaction in behavior therapy: Development and first application of an observational system. *British Journal of Clinical Psychology, 28,* 213–226.

Schutz, W. C. (1973). Encounter. In R. Corsini (Ed.), *Current psychotherapies.* Itasca, Ill: Peacock.

Seamans, J. H. (1956). Premature ejaculation: A new approach. *Southern Medical Journal, 49,* 353–357.

Seligman, M. E. P. (1975). *Helplessness.* San Francisco: Freeman.

Seligman, M. E. P., Abramson, L. Y., Semmel, A., & von Baeyer, C. (1979). Depressive attributional style. *Journal of Abnormal Psychology, 88,* 242–247.

Sells, S. B. (Ed.) (1963). *Stimulus determinants of behavior.* New York: Ronald.

Shahar, A., & Merbaum, M. (1981). The interaction between subject characteristics and self-control procedures in the treatment of interpersonal anxiety. *Cognitive Therapy and Research, 5,* 221–224.

Shapiro, D. H., Jr. (1978). *Precision nirvana.* Englewood Cliffs, NJ: Prentice-Hall.

Shectman, F. A. (1975). Operant conditioning and psychoanalysis: Contrasts, similarities, and some thoughts about integration. *American Journal of Psychotherapy, 29,* 72–78.

Shoham-Solomon, V., Avner, R., & Neeman, R. (1989). You've changed if you do and changed if you don't: Mechanisms underlying paradoxial interventions. *Journal of Consulting and Clinical Psychology, 57,* 590–598.

Shostrom, E. L. (Producer). (1986). *Three approaches to psychotherapy: III* (film). Corona Del Mar, CA: Psychological and Educational Films.

Silberschatz, G., Fretter, P., & Curtis, J. (1986). How do interpretations influence the process of psychotherapy? *Journal of Consulting and Clinical Psychology, 54,* 646–652.

Silverman, L. H. (1974). Some psychoanalytic considerations of non-psychanalytic therapies: On the possibility of integrating treatment approaches and related issues. *Psychotherapy: Theory, Research, and Practice, 11,* 298–305.

Singer, J. L. (1988). Reinterpreting the transference. In D. C. Turk & P. Salovey (Eds.) *Reasoning, interference, and judgment in clinical psychology* (pp. 182–205). New York: Free.

Singer, J. A., & Salovey, P. (1988). Mood and memory: Evaluating the network theory of affect. *Clinical Psychology Review, 8,* 211–251.

Sloane, R. B. (1969). The converging paths of behavior therapy and psychotherapy. *American Journal of Psychiatry, 125,* 877–885.

Smith, M. L., Glass, G. V., & Miller, T. I. (1980). *The benefits of psychotherapy.* Baltimore: Johns Hopkins University Press.

Smith, T. W. (1982). Irrational beliefs in the cause and treatment of emotional distress: A critical review of the rational-emotive model. *Clinical Psychology Review, 2,* 505–522.

Snyder, W. U. (1950). Clinical methods: Psychotherapy. *Annual Review of Psychology, 1*, 221-234.

Staats, A. W., & Staats, C. K. (1963). *Complex human behavior.* New York: Holt, Rinehart, & Winston.

Stanton, H. R., & Litwak, E. (1955). Toward the development of a short form Test of Interpersonal Competence. *American Sociological Review, 20*, 668-674.

Strupp, H. H. (1967). What is psychotherapy? *Contemporary Psychology, 12*, 41-42.

Strupp, H. H. (1973a). Foreword in D. J. Kiesler, *The process of psychotherapy.* Chicago: Aldine.

Strupp, H. H. (1973b). On the basic ingredients of psychotherapy. *Journal of Consulting and Clinical Psychology, 41*, 1-8.

Strupp, H.H. (1976). Some critical comments on the future of psychoanalytic therapy. *Bulletin of the Menninger Clinic, 40*, 238-254.

Strupp, H. H. (1978). *Are psychoanalytic therapists beginning to practice cognitive behavior therapy or is behavior therapy turning psychoanalytic?* Presented at symposium, clinical-cognitive theory of psychotherapy, American Psychological Association, Toronto.

Strupp, H. H. (1988). What is therapeutic change? *Journal of Cognitive Psychotherapy, 2*, 75-82.

Strupp, H. H., & Binder, J. (1984). *Psychotherapy in a new key.* New York: Plenum.

Sullivan, H. S. (1954). *The psychiatric interview.* New York: Norton.

Sundberg, N. D., & Tyler, L. E. (1962). *Clinical psychology.* New York: Appleton-Century-Crofts.

Sutton-Simon, K., & Goldfried, M. R. (1982). *Cognitive processes in social anxiety.* Unpublished manuscript, Oberlin College.

Szasz, T. S. (1961). *The myth of mental illness.* New York: Hoeber.

Taylor, S. E., & Crocker, J. (1981). Schematic bases of social information processing. In E. T. Higgins, P. Hermann, & M. P. Zanna (Eds.), *The Ontario symposium on personality and social psychology* (Vol. 1). Hillsdale, NJ: Erlbaum.

Thomas, L. F., & Harri-Augstein, E. S. (1985). *Self-organized learning: Foundation of a conversational science for psychology.* London: Routledge & Kegan Paul.

Thoresen, C. E. (1973). Behavioral humanism. In C. E. Thoresen (Ed.), *Behavior modification in education.* Chicago: University of Chicago Press.

Thoresen, C. E., & Coates, T. J. (1978). What does it mean to be a behavior therapist? *Counseling Psychologist, 7*, 3-21.

Thoresen, C. E., & Mahoney, M. J. (1974). *Behavioral self-control.* New York: Holt, Rinehart, & Winston.

Thorndyke, P. W., & Hayes-Roth, B. (1979). The use of schemata in the acquisition and transfer of knowledge. *Cognitive Psychology, 11*, 2-106.

Thorne, F. C. (1950). Principles of personality counseling. Brandon, VT: *Journal of Clinical Psychology.*

Thorpe, J. G., & Schmidt, E. (1963). Therapeutic failure in a case of aversion therapy. *Behaviour Research and Therapy, 1,* 293-296.

Torrey, E. F. (1972). What Western psychotherapies can learn from witchdoctors. *American Journal of Orthopsychiatry, 42,* 69-71.

Truax, C. B., & Mitchell, K. M. (1971). Research on certain therapist interpersonal skills in relation to process and outcome. In A. E. Bergin & S. L. Garfield (Eds.), *Handbook on psychotherapy and behavior change* (pp. 299-344). New York: Wiley.

Tulving, E. (1972). Episodic and semantic memory. In E. Tulving & W. Donaldson (Eds.), *Organization of memory.* New York: Academic Press.

Turner, R. M. (1993). Dynamic cognitive-behavior therapy. In T. Giles (Ed.), *Handbook of effective psychotherapy.* New York: Plenum.

Tversky, A., & Kahnemann, D. (1974). Judgment under uncertainty: Heuristics and biases. *Science, 185,* 1124-1131.

Ullmann, L. P., & Krasner, L. (Eds.) (1965). *Case studies in behavior modification.* New York: Holt, Rinehart, & Winston.

Wachtel, P. L. (1973). On fact, hunch, and stereotype: A reply to Mischel. *Journal of Abnormal Psychology, 82,* 537-540.

Wachtel, P. L. (1975). Behavior therapy and the facilitation of psychoanalytic exploration. *Psychotherapy: Theory, Research, and Practice, 12,* 68-72.

Wachtel, P. L. (1977). *Psychoanalysis and behavior therapy: Toward an integration.* New York: Basic Books.

Wachtel, P. L. (1980). Investigation and its discontents: Some constraints on progress in psychological research. *American Psychologist, 35,* 399-408.

Wachtel, P. L. (1981). Transference, schema, and assimilation: The relevance of Piaget to the psychoanalytic theory of transference. In Chicago Institute for Psychoanalysis (Eds.), *Annual of Psychoanalysis* (Vol. 8). New York: International Universities Press.

Wachtel, P. L. (1985). Need for theory. *International Newsletter of Paradigmatic Psychology, I,* 15-17.

Wachtel, P. L., & McKinney, M. (1992). Cyclical psychodynamics. In J. C. Norcross and M. R. Goldfried (Eds.), *Handbook of psychotherapy integration.* New York: Basic Books.

Wallace, J. (1966). An abilities conception of personality: Some implications for personality measurement. *American Psychologist, 21,* 132-138.

Wallace, J. (1967). What units shall we employ? Allport's question revisited. *Journal of Consulting Psychology, 31,* 56-64.

Wallace, J., & Sechrest, L. (1963). Frequency hypothesis and content analysis of projective techniques. *Journal of Consulting Psychology, 27,* 387-393.

Wandersman, A., Poppen, P. J., & Ricks, D. F. (Eds.) (1976). *Humanism and behaviorism: Dialogue and growth.* Elmford, NY: Pergamon.

Watson, G. (1940). Areas of agreement in psychotherapy. *American Journal of Orthopsychiatry, 10,* 698–709.

Weinberg, R., Gould, D., & Jackson, A. (1979). Expectations and performance: An empirical test of Bandura's self-efficacy theory. *Journal of Sport Psychology, 1,* 320–331.

Weiss, R.L. (1968). Operant conditioning techniques in psychological assessment. In P. McRynolds (Ed.), *Advances in psychological assessment.* Palo Alto, CA: Science and Behavior Books.

Weiss, R. L. (1980). Strategic behavioral marital therapy: Toward a model for assessment and intervention. *Advances in Family Intervention: Assessment and Theory, 1,* 229–271.

Weiss, J., & Sampson, H. (1986). *The psychoanalytic process.* New York: Guilford.

Weitzman, B. (1967). Behavior therapy and psychotherapy. *Psychological Review, 74,* 300–317.

Werner, H. (1948). *Comparative psychology of mental development* (Rev. ed.) Chicago: Follett.

Westen, D. (1988). Transference and information processing. *Clinical Psychology Review, 8,* 161–179.

Westen, D. (1991). Social cognition and object relations. *Psychological Bulletin, 109,* 429–455.

Wheeler, W. M. (1949). An analysis of Rorschach indices of male homosexuality. *Rorschach Research Exchange, 13,* 97–126.

Wheelis, A. (1973). *How people change.* New York: Harper & Row.

White, R. W. (1959). Motivation re-considered: The concept of competence. *Psychological Review, 66,* 297–333.

Whitehouse, F. A. (1967). The concept of therapy: A review of some essentials. *Rehabilitation Literature, 28,* 238–247.

Wilson, G. T. (1978). The importance of being theoretical: A commentary on Bandura's "Self-efficacy: Towards a unifying theory of behavioral change." *Advances in Behaviour Research and Therapy, 1,* 217–230.

Wilson, G. T. (1982). Psychotherapy process and procedure: The behavioral mandate. *Behavior Therapy, 13,* 291–312.

Wilson, G. T. (1990). Clinical issues and strategies in the practice of behavior therapy. In C. M. Franks, G. T. Wilson, P. C. Kendall, & J. P. Foreyt (Eds.), *Review of behavior therapy, (Vol. 12, pp. 271–301).* New York: Guilford Press.

Wilson, G. T., & Davison, G. C. (1971). Processes of fear reduction in systematic desensitization: Animal studies. *Psychological Bulletin, 76,* 1–14.

Wise, E. H., & Haynes, S. N. (1983). Cognitive treatment of test anxiety: Rational restructuring versus attentional training. *Cognitive Therapy Research, 7,* 69–78.

Wolf, E. (1966). Learning theory and psychoanalysis. *British Journal of Medical Psychology, 39,* 1-10.

Wolfe, B. E. (October 1983). *Behavior therapy researchers: Should they study non-behavioral therapies.* Paper presented at the meeting of the Association for Advancement of Behavior Therapy, Washington, DC.

Wolfe, B. E., & Goldfried, M. R. (1988). Research on psychotherapy integration: Recommendations and conclusions from an NIMH workshop. *Journal of Consulting and Clinical Psychology, 56,* 448-451.

Wolpe, J. (1958). *Psychotherapy by reciprocal inhibition.* Stanford, CA: Stanford University Press.

Wolpe, J. (1964). The systematic desensitization treatment of neuroses. In H. J. Eysenck (Ed.), *Experiments in behaviour therapy* (pp. 21-39). New York: Macmillan.

Wolpe, J. (1973).*The practice of behavior therapy* (2nd ed.). New York: Pergamon Press.

Wolpe, J. (1978). Self-efficacy theory and psychotherapeutic change: A square peg for a round hole. *Andvances in Behaviour Research and Therapy, 1,* 231-236.

Wolpe, J., & Lang, P. J. (1964). A fear survey schedule for use in behavior therapy. *Behaviour Research and Therapy, 2,* 27-30.

Wolpe, J., & Lazarus, A. A. (1966). *Behaviour therapy techniques.* Elmsford, NY: Pergamon Press.

Woody, R. H. (1968). Toward a rationale for psychobehavioral therapy. *Archives of General Psychiatry, 19,* 197-204.

Woody, R. H. (1971).*Psychobehavioral counseling and therapy: Integrating behavioral and insight techniques.* New York: Appleton-Century-Crofts.

Woody, R. H. (1973). Integrated aversion therapy and psychotherapy: Two sexual deviation case studies. *Journal of Sex Research, 9,* 313-324.

Wright, J., & Sabourin, S. (1987). Les contributions du modele behavioral a la problematique du rapprochement en psychotherapie. In C. Lecomte & L. G. Castonguay (Eds.), *Rapprochement et integration en psychotherapie: Psychoanalyse, behaviorisme et humanisme* (pp. 81-100). Chicoutimi (Qc): Gaetan Morin editeur.

Young, J., & Swift, W. (1988). Schema-focused cognitive therapy for personality disorders: Part I. *International Cognitive Therapy Newsletter, 4,* 13-14.

Zeisset, R. M. (1968). Desensitization and relaxation in the modification of psychiatric patients' interview behavior. *Journal of Abnormal Psychology, 73,* 18-24.

Zigler, E., & Phillips, L. (1961). Psychiatric diagnosis: A critique. *Journal of Abnormal and Social Psychology, 63,* 607-618.

Name Index

Subject Index

BEHAVIOR THERAPY IN PSYCHIATRIC HOSPITALS

**Patrick Corrigan, PsyD, and
Robert Paul Liberman, MD, Editors**

This volume provides practical guidelines for implementing behavior therapy programs, overcoming administrative and clinical obstacles, and maintaining quality care in psychiatric settings. These programs are intended to complement the judicious use of psychopharmacological agents in treatment.

Contents:

Overview of Behavior Therapy in Therapeutic Environments, *P. Corrigan and R.P. Liberman* • The Clinical Research Unit at Camarillo State Hospital, *S.M. Glynn, et al.* • The Transitional Unit of the Albuquerque VA Medical Center, *R. Hierholzer and M. Thornbrough* • The Social Learning Program at the Forensic Unit of Fulton State Hospital, *A.A. Menditto, et al.* • Obstacles in the Implementation of a Behavior Therapy Ward in a State Psychiatric Hospital, *H. Franco and R. Kelly* • The Behavior Therapy Program at the Extended Care Unit of Tinley Park Mental Health Center, *P.W. Corrigan, et al.*

• Evolution of Behavior Therapy in a Changing Mental Institution: The Behavior Therapy Unit at the Haar Psychiatric Hospital, *F. Mohrs, et al.* • A Behavioral Medicine Unit in a University Hospital, *L. Dahlgren, et al.* • Cognitive Behavior Therapy for Neurotic Disorders, *P. Levendusky, et al.* • Behavior Therapy in the Residential Treatment of Children and Adolescents, *G. Moss* • Factors Affecting the Implementation, Delivery and Durability of Behavior Therapy in Psychiatric Hospitals, *R.P. Liberman and P. Corrigan* • Selling Behavioral Technology in the Healthcare Market Place, *G. Moss*

Springer Series: Behavior Therapy
1994   288pp   0-8261-8480-4   *hardcover*

536 Broadway, New York, NY 10012-3955 • (212) 431-4370 • Fax (212) 941-7842